T0315441

PRAISE FOR *UNEXPECTED*

"In this new book, *Unexpected: Finding Resilience through Functional Medicine, Science, and Faith*, Dr. Jill Carnahan shares her riveting personal story and uses her shocking diagnosis with aggressive breast cancer at twenty-five-years-old to introduce a new paradigm for readers, where fear and the unknown are replaced with resilience, healing, and a very realistic set of tools to inspire health and communication with those who deal in health."

> – **DR. MARK HYMAN,** author of fourteen *New York Times* Bestsellers including *The Pegan Diet* and *Food Fix*

"Dr. Jill Carnahan shares her decades of work in clinical practice and walks you through exactly how to use the right tools in the right ways to make your body work the way you choose. You will rarely find a book where a well-qualified doctor exposes her own medical journey for all to see. Prepare to be inspired and informed when you set this precious book down."

> – **DAVE ASPREY,** father of Biohacking, founder of Bulletproof, and *New York Times* Bestseller

"*Unexpected* is a beautiful snapshot into the world of a young woman facing a life-altering diagnosis in the form of an aggressive breast cancer at only twenty-five-years-old. Dr. Jill Carnahan shares her journey with all of us in the hopes that her experience as a patient will help prepare us to fight the unconventional and eventually change how we communicate with those in healthcare. What a read!"

> – **JOAN LUNDEN,** journalist, author, television host, and cohost of ABC's *Good Morning America* from 1980 to 1997

"Dr. Jill Carnahan's *Unexpected* is one of the few books that guides practitioners and patients through the ups and downs of traveling the health highway—speed bumps, detours, flat tires, and all. Dr. Carnahan is a master storyteller, and this book is a powerful glimpse into her own story, and it is loaded with important protocols from the unexpectedly compassionate and inspiring MD."

> – **DR. AMY MYERS,** *New York Times* Bestselling Author

"Dr. Jill Carnahan's book, *Unexpected*, uses her personal story to create a powerful road map for any reader who has had to face a chronic health condition. It is a guidebook that is loaded with resources to empower patients with new tools to support their journeys—and to know how to communicate with their doctors to encourage a more holistic and partnered approach to root-cause healing."

– **DR. FRANK LIPMAN,** chief medical officer of The Well,
founder of Eleven Eleven Wellness, and bestselling author

"Dr. Carnahan is both a clinical master and an amazing human spirit who brings the best of her years of experience as a true doctor and healer to her book, *Unexpected*. Through her own personal experience with environmental illness and the successful management of thousands of patients with unexpected chronic illnesses, she lays out a blueprint for the creation of health. This is a must-read for anyone seeking answers on how to manage complex health issues."

– **DR. JEFFREY BLAND,** FACN, FACB, CNS, functional
medicine thought leader, and cofounder of the Institute for
Functional Medicine

"This is a must-read, inspiring, life-altering book. Unlike the experiences so many of us have with our doctors, Dr. Jill Carnahan is not distant, aloof, or hiding behind her intellect as an MD. She leads with a brave transparency, sharing her compellingly told story as a breast cancer patient with a powerfully kind heart."

– **DR. TERRY WAHLS,** FACP, IFMCP, and bestselling author
of *The Wahls Protocol: A Radical New Way to Treat All Chronic
Autoimmune Conditions Using Paleo Principles*

"Dr. Jill Carnahan, like this book, is a light to the world. Her story is one of perseverance, love, and above all, grace. She has been given the extraordinary gift of finding hope for people who are hurting, especially herself."

– **RORY FEEK (JOEY+RORY),** Grammy-winning music artist,
and bestselling author

"In this new book, *Unexpected: Finding Resilience through Functional Medicine, Science, and Faith*, Dr. Jill Carnahan shares her riveting personal story and uses her shocking diagnosis with aggressive breast cancer at twenty-five to introduce a new paradigm for readers, where fear and the unknown are replaced with resilience, healing, and a very realistic set of tools to inspire health and communication with those who work in healthcare. A must read for those dealing with complex, chronic illnesses looking for innovative ways to heal."

> **– DR. RICHARD HOROWITZ,** *New York Times* Best Selling Author of *Why Can't I Get Better: Solving the Mystery of Lyme and Chronic Disease*

"*Unexpected* is the deeply personal story of Dr. Jill Carnahan's compelling life-journey. You will immediately sense her compassion and genuine desire to give people hope to feel vibrant again. After facing her own journey through a life-threatening illness, Dr. Jill used her experiences as a powerful force in shaping her passion for teaching others how to heal and thrive. Every word in this powerful book leaves you with an incredible sense of hope and desire to not only want to live, but also to fall in love with life itself."

> **– IZABELLA WENTZ,** PharmD, FASCP, and *New York Times* Bestselling Author of *Hashimoto's Protocol: A 90-Day Plan for Reversing Thyroid Symptoms and Getting Your Life Back*

"*Unexpected* is a deeply personal story of Dr. Jill Carnahan's compelling life journey. It exemplifies her resilience and innate ability to transform vulnerability into courage. Dr. Jill has truly carried the cross to help the world find infinite health. You will immediately sense her compassion, genuine desire to give people hope that they can feel safe in sickness, and ability to promote wellbeing, no matter what the situation. Dr. Jill 's experience is a powerful force in shaping functional medicine and in the teaching of others so her knowledge lives forever. Every word in this powerful book made me feel more alive and reminded me that those of us who heal need to share our gifts for the benefit of others."

> **– DR. CHAD J. PRUSMACK,** MD FAANS, IFMPC, chief of neurosurgery Rocky Mountain Spine Clinic, neurosurgical consultant to the Denver Broncos and the United States Olympic Team, founder of Resilience Code

"This book is a glimpse into Dr. Jill Carnahan's story of becoming the patient and facing a life-altering illness. It is a glimpse of her fighting for her health and overcoming sickness and skeptics by using both science and faith. And if that wasn't enough, she also offers practical advice and resources to help patients discover powerful new health modalities in functional and alternative medicine. I loved every word in this inspirational and deeply personal book."

> – **DR. PAMELA W. SMITH,** MPH, MS, founder of the Fellowship in Anti-Aging and Regenerative Medicine

"I couldn't put it down! If you're feeling the constraints of your health issues, Dr. Carnahan will transform your life with easy-to-implement medical tips and a renewed sense of faith and resilience. The author will make you laugh and cry while exciting you with the possibility that an extraordinary existence awaits you. No matter how dark or difficult your health circumstances are, Dr. Jill will encourage and empower you. This was one fascinating read! This beautifully written book should be a required reading for all medical doctors!"

> – **SUZY COHEN,** RPh, syndicated columnist, and author of *Drug Muggers*

"I am thrilled to give five stars to Dr. Jill Carnahan's book, *Unexpected: Finding Resilience through Functional Medicine, Science, and Faith.* Dr. Jill is a brilliant clinician, and her book should be read by every medical student in any realm of health, as well as anyone struggling with a health crisis. She is providing a lifestyle Rx—simplifying sophisticated mechanisms into everyday language. This book is a must read!"

> – **DR. MADIHA SAEED,** bestselling author

"As a Naturopathic Doctor, I believe Dr. Jill Carnahan has done a remarkable job painting a clear picture of what a serious health crisis looks and feels like from the patient's point of view and loaded it with protocols and tools that are inspiringly simple and effective wrapped around her deeply personal story. This book will change your life."

> – **DR. DARIN INGELS,** FAAEM, bestselling author of *The Lyme Solution*

"Jill Carnahan's new book can be a reference manual for healthcare practitioners, as well as a roadmap to guide any of us toward the health we deserve. In *Unexpected*, she masterfully integrates decades of clinical experience as an MD with an unflinchingly honest account of what she went through after being diagnosed with a very aggressive form of breast cancer in her early twenties while she was in medical school. Her raw and honest account of her own journey reminds us that this is not the dress rehearsal."

> **– DR. KELLY MCCANN,** ABOIM diplomate and renowned mast cell activation expert

"In this inspiring book, Dr. Jill Carnahan shares the story of her incredible journey, revealing how her deep faith set the stage for a transformative journey that enabled her to defy expectations and survive a brutal diagnosis of aggressive breast cancer at only twenty-five. She was able to chart a lifelong course filled with meaning and purpose and inspire a new level of patient care. Whether you're struggling with your own health obstacles, looking to improve your life, or seeking inspiration as a health practitioner. Dr. Jill's story will give you the inspiration and tools you need."

> **– DR. RAND MCCLAIN,** chief medical officer at Live Cell Research and Regenerative Sports Medicine, and author of *Cheating Death: The New Science of Living Longer and Better*

"This is a must-read book. Dr. Jill Carnahan not only shares her journey through breast cancer, Crohn's, and mold toxicity, but thoroughly explains how the modern medicine approach needs to change too. She also guides patients to be more proactive in their own healthcare. I appreciated the practical tips and resources she gives us while weaving them in between her heartfelt stories of sadness and triumph. All who are struggling with health issues will find it both helpful and relatable on so many levels. I absolutely loved it from start to finish!"

> **– DR. CARRIE JONES,** FABNE, MPH, and author at DUTCH Test

"I read Dr. Jill Carnahan's entire book cover to cover in one plane ride from Phoenix to New Jersey! I couldn't put it down and absolutely loved it on so many levels. It is loaded with fabulous functional medicine information and beautiful life lessons that I believe will transform the reader. This is a very special book!"

> – **MARGIE BISSINGER,** PT, integrative health coach, and happiness trainer

"It used to be my limited view that as long as we get the right nutrition, supplements, some sleep, and movement, there is no stopping us to heal and thrive. Dr. Jill, through her own life stories and empathetic encounters of her patients, paints a much more complete picture to healing—one where faith, love, empathy, forgiveness, and intuition are just as critical to our healing."

> – **MAGDALENA WSZELAKI,** bestselling author of *Overcoming Estrogen Dominance* and *Cooking for Hormone Balance*

"A brilliant functional medicine doctor tells you all her wisdom about the journey from deathly ill to healthy and happy in a homey, approachable way. Practical checklists, wise perspectives, and the steps to fix the health issues draining you and dragging you down keep this book both a fast-paced read and an ongoing resource for what to do to feel your vitality again."

> – **SUSAN BRATTON,** CEO and co-founder of Personal Life Media, Inc.

Unexpected

FINDING RESILIENCE
THROUGH FUNCTIONAL MEDICINE,
SCIENCE, AND FAITH

DR. JILL CARNAHAN, MD

Forefront
BOOKS

Published by Forefront Books.

Library of Congress Control Number: 2022915941

Print ISBN: 978-1-63763-095-2
E-book ISBN: 978-1-63763-096-9

Cover Design by Bruce Gore, Gore Studio, Inc.
Interior Design by Bill Kersey, KerseyGraphics

Incurable doesn't mean healing is not possible. It simply

means there is not a drug that reverses the condition.

—Dr. Jill Carnahan

Acknowledgements

I WOULD LIKE TO EXPRESS MY DEEPEST GRATITUDE FOR THE LOVE and support of each person who accompanied me in the journey of writing and publishing this book and especially the Forefront publishing team and TGC.

Thank you to Topher, my writing coach, who encouraged me when I felt like giving up, who kept me afloat when life got crazy, and who taught me how to climb mountains.

I am extremely grateful for Ali, Natalie, Jessica and Loretta, my indispensable office staff, who kept my busy medical clinic afloat while I was seeing patients, writing this book and producing a documentary. And to each of the beautiful women who offer their healing services at the Flatiron Functional Medicine Office: Rene, JoEllen, Haley, Megan, Judy, Nicole, and Crystal, together our healing potential is limitless.

My unconditional love to each of my precious friends who are quick to respond when I need a hike at Mt. Sanitas, a coloring session, a coffee break, or just a prayer: Ilene Naomi, Shelese, Christine, Sarah, Suzy, Sheryl, Ashley, Cheryl, Susie, Claire, Suzanne, Ann, Tammy, Lauryn, Conan, and many others.

To the coffee shops who kept me alert with coconut milk lattes and San Pellegrino during my long writing sessions, I raise my cup to you: Brewing Market, Bittersweet Cafe, and Cavegirl Coffee.

I continue to be forever grateful to my many brilliant professional colleagues who have been guests on my podcast, shared my blog articles, attended my lectures, and encouraged me in ways too numerous to count!

Thank you Daffnee, Kyle, and Peter, my gifted and loyal marketing team for believing in me and very special thanks for Mary Agnes and Viral Integrity Team for managing the book launch process.

To the talented glam squad who brings out the best in me— Heather, Gwen, Kianna, and Laura Rose

To my loving supportive parents, Ken and Kathy, my siblings, Jeff, Jason, Jamie, and Jeremy and their spouses, my stepdaughters Heather and Candice and the inspirational, beloved matriarch of my family, Grandma Farney, my true hero.

To Dan and Aaron of Embark Features, who filmed and encouraged me in the making of the documentary *Doctor/Patient* while I was writing this book and especially to Phil, our generous executive producer, my deepest gratitude for supporting us in the project.

And to my source of strength and support, love and laughter, and adventure, DW.

Foreword

by Sara Gottfried, MD

WHEN I MET JILL CARNAHAN, M.D., I KNEW IMMEDIATELY THAT WE would be fast friends and soul mates. Yes, we are close in age. Yes, we are colleagues in integrative and functional medicine. Yes, we are both obsessed with our mission to lessen the suffering of the people we serve. But perhaps more importantly, we both faced challenges early in our careers with health issues that mainstream medicine couldn't resolve. It led us to question the dogma of mainstream medicine and look for answers beyond the usual silos of disease-based care. We are physicians who want you to avoid unnecessary suffering with your own health issues, but we are also humans searching for purpose and meaning in all that we do. As we healed from our challenges, we built the type of medical practices that we most needed ourselves as patients, and it created an unshakable bond between us that we will share throughout our lifetimes.

Another commonality is that Dr. Jill and I were entrenched in a high-performance, success-driven, science-based healthcare system that continues to be more focused on putting you into a diagnostic box and offering a pharmaceutical and less focused on the body-based, intuitive approach to healing. In fact, the grueling hours of medical training and emotional trauma of having patients on the edge of death may make some physicians more disembodied, robotic, and emotionally unavailable.

I've learned most of us need both: care that is evidence-based but grounded in love. And that is what Dr. Jill offers you.

When we first met in person at a medical conference five years ago, I had listened to Dr. Jill's podcasts about mold and other toxic environmental exposures, hitting the rewind more times than I can count. At the time, I was desperate to understand how mold exposure might be disrupting my hormones and those of my patients. Dr. Jill has a facility with complex topics that makes me swoon intellectually, but under all the knowledge and experience, she is a true healer brimming with love. Maybe you've noticed that a lot of today's physician healers are wounded. Not Jill. It's the combination of knowledge and wholeness that won me over, and it will win you over too.

I've observed in my 25 years of practicing medicine that the people who've experienced the greatest hardships—fighting cancer at a young age, dealing with an incurable autoimmune condition, or getting exposed to toxic stress from environmental chemicals, mold, or trauma—often become the most soulful, compassionate, gifted healers and mystics, searching for deeper truths. They are the people who tend to buck convention, so it's rare to find them at your local hospital or clinic.

Why does trauma create healers and mystics? While it may be hard to explain on a purely scientific basis, we can look at genetics as an example. In my precision medicine practice, I see patients daily who are born with genetic variations that create problems like impairments in detoxification, inability to make sufficient brain neurotransmitters, or predispositions to making more inflammatory chemicals in the body. These genetic variations, especially when a patient has many of them, add up to feeling unwell or struggling with symptoms that fly below the radar of your well-meaning primary care doctor. What I've noticed is that the people who have the worst genetic blueprint are paradoxically the most resilient in the face of adversity. They know how to adapt and thrive, because they are very practiced at it, cells to soul. Whether conscious or not, one's ability to adapt to challenges and grow from trauma may be our greatest opportunity for health and healing. These patients who have suffered, overcome difficult odds, and have been told that there is nothing wrong or nothing else to be done, go on to become the mystics, the seers, and the teachers, showing others the direction we need to go to become whole.

My name is Dr. Sara Gottfried, M.D. I am a Harvard-educated medical doctor, scientist, researcher, teacher, and author of four *New York Times* bestselling books. Like Dr. Jill, I have been practicing integrative, functional, and precision medicine for many decades. In the process, I have become adept at doing thorough examinations of physical and genetic profiles (called phenotyping) of patients, helping them heal, not only from genetic and biochemical imbalances, but also from the more mysterious aspects of environmental exposures, toxicity, relationships, and traumas that impact the patient's health. When you stop reaching for pharmaceuticals to mask your symptoms—popping sleeping pills, pain killers, or anti-anxiety medications—you open up an entirely new world of possibility, prevention, healing, and repair, as Dr. Jill shows you in this book.

As you get to know Dr. Jill on these pages, you too will sense that she is a kindred soul. She has weathered many difficult life experiences but has emerged in a way that is extraordinary and inspiring. Many people experience traumatic stress, and it leaves them with a victim mindset. They become filled with doubt and fear, as if the world is out to get them. On the other hand, there are those rare people who go through suffering and emerge with greater trust in humanity, a profound faith in the divine, a brighter light, deep, abiding love, and trust in the universe. That's what you feel when you meet Dr. Jill.

Using her gift of compassionate wisdom, born through experience, she brings us *Unexpected*, the story of her own journey of healing and finding resilience through functional medicine, science, and faith—a story that will inspire and transform you.

In her book, she bridges the science-based, "quantitative" side of medicine with the more grace-filled space of love, connection, and finding meaning no matter what you are traversing, allowing the greatest possible transformation and healing. Her book reads as if you were sitting with her over a cup of tea in a riveting conversation, a nourishing treat for your soul. Through the pages, you will feel her deep presence and understanding born from her most painful life experiences to be the best map for your own journey.

I've learned that deep presence becomes deep medicine for the reader as you follow her remarkable story and guidance. She will take you from her life as a child growing up on a corn and soybean farm in Central Illinois to the shocking diagnosis of cancer at twenty-five years old while immersed in medical school, to a label of incurable autoimmune disease, and finally to a battle with environmental toxicity and mold nearly a decade later that brought her to her knees in surrender. By far the most painful and shocking transformation came after her husband walked out after twenty years and she was left to grapple with her own identity and self-worth, learning for the first time to truly love herself in the process. In the final chapter, you will discover the most powerful healing lesson of all. Although each chapter details the ways she found resilience and healing, the last chapter reveals the power of unconditional love, which she found by trusting her own innate wisdom and intuition, applying self-love and compassion to transmute past trauma into fuel for resilience, and developing a shining new purpose to help others transform their lives as well.

Dr. Jill provides a new beacon of hope and tenderness as we face any obstacle. She and I were destined to teach, build bridges, and bring compassion, heart, and coherence back to the practice of medicine. Please know and trust that your grief and struggle can be transformed into something bigger and profound. You have taken the reins by reaching for her book, and you will find so much hope and healing in these pages. Maybe one day our world will come to understand that unconditional love and connection are the foundation of all healing.

Sara Gottfried, MD
Berkeley, California

Contents

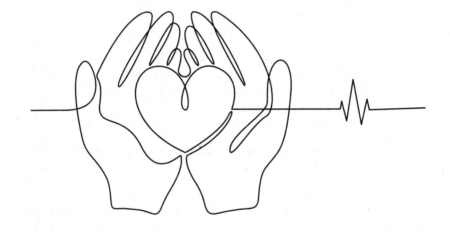

Be Open to the Unexpected

MY CLINIC HAD A THREE-YEAR WAIT LIST WHEN ALEX HUDSON'S mother called my office. I'll never forget my receptionist's words: "Her mom said that she doesn't have three months, let alone three years."

"Call her back and get her on the schedule," I told her. "Let's see if we can help her."

As I reviewed Alex's records, my heart sank. The symptoms of mast cell activation syndrome (MCAS) and inflammation were the most severe I'd ever seen. Due to her genetics, underlying infections, toxic overload, and myriad other factors, her immune system had triggered an exaggerated inflammatory response that was destroying her health from the inside out. Her symptoms were so severe that her gastrointestinal tract was rejecting all but a handful of foods, and she was in critical condition due to severe malnutrition. When Alex and her mother flew out to Colorado from California for the appointment, they had already seen nearly forty doctors in their search for answers. Only in her early twenties, Alex was declining rapidly.

Although I am never one to give up hope, it was clear to me at the first visit that any attempt at healing would be a long shot. There was no medication or supplement I could prescribe that would act quickly enough to reverse the damage to her gut or the ranging immune inflammation at this late stage, but I was willing to try. Alex was literally wasting away before her family's eyes.

After reviewing her entire medical history and doing a physical exam, I sat in my office, looking across the desk at Alex and her mother. My mind tried to find the right words and my heart pounded as I fought back my emotions. I began flipping through her chart again, thinking maybe there was something I had missed. As they waited for my summary of findings, I saw the words I needed. At my clinic, one of the questions I ask every new patient on the admission form is, "What is your source of strength?" Alex had written, "My faith in God." I stopped flipping through the chart. Maybe there was something I could do.

I asked Alex and her mom, "With your permission, may I pray for you?"

I reached across my desk and grabbed each of their hands, making a circle, and said a prayer for Alex: "Divine Father, sometimes you lead us to a place where it seems all hope is lost. Despite all appearances to the contrary, I believe that each of our difficult experiences still contain blessings, and today I pray that, in some way, you would show this precious daughter an unexpected miracle, the grace that comes when we see no tangible way out of our suffering. I pray that you would give her peace, infuse her life with meaning and purpose in whatever time she has left, and relieve her suffering and pain."

Twenty-three years earlier, Alex had been born into a vibrant and active family. Besides her older brother, Garrett, her golden retriever (aptly named Buddy) was her constant companion. She loved spending time with her family and excelled in many school sports, including softball, volleyball, cheerleading, and track. She was not only athletically talented but excelled in school as well. By the time she graduated high school, she was awarded a full-ride scholarship to UCLA. Her future would have been bright had it not been for the devastating diagnosis of Lyme disease and MCAS.

When eleven-year-old Alex complained that her legs hurt, her mother, Jody, thought it was just growing pains, but in the ten years that followed, Alex perplexed dozens of conventional doctors with her symptoms and was considered a "medical mystery" until she was finally given the appropriate diagnosis. By then it was too late. Even after the pain became so severe that she became bedridden, she never lost her joyful spirit and desire to help others. At Christmastime she would often return her own gifts to buy clothing, socks, or other necessities for the homeless. "She was never focused on her own suffering," her mother said. "She was always thinking more of how she could help others, even in the end."

Alex was able to spend the last months of her life at home with her beloved family. As her physical body continued to decline, she was unable to eat and had to get nutrition through an IV, but she found unexpected meaning and purpose in her last days. She cast a vision with her mother to create a foundation whose mission would be to increase research efforts for Lyme disease and MCAS and also provide financial support for patients' testing and treatment. She hoped that by supporting earlier intervention and diagnosis, she might help prevent others from her own fate of floundering as a "medical mystery" for ten long years before she was correctly diagnosed. The vision of helping to increase awareness of these complex and chronic illnesses grew into the Alex Hudson Lyme Foundation and the memoir written by her mother, *My Promise to Alex*.

Years later, Alex's mother summarized her visit with me: "Dr. Jill wasn't able to help Alex medically, but she helped both of us to see that there are other types of healing, including emotional and spiritual. Her encouragement and compassion awakened Alex to find her deeper purpose, which transcended life itself."

I would much rather talk about the many patients I've helped overcome disease and go on to live long and healthy lives, but Alex's story best exemplifies what this book, and my life, are all about: positive transformation against all odds.

This book is written for those times in life when you feel as if you're all alone, floating in uncertainty and you don't know quite where to turn for answers.

My own journey is about finding resilience when I least expected it and overcoming my difficulties through functional medicine, science, and faith. Although my journey is unique, so is yours. Even if you don't share my spiritual beliefs, there is a powerful message in the transcendence we can find when in the middle of the darkness if we stay open to the unexpected.

Alex helped me realize that no matter how much I want to heal every patient who comes to see me, sometimes there are no medical answers. What I can offer is unconditional love and encouragement for each person to find meaning and purpose through their own journey. Alex found her greater mission in creating a foundation that would outlive her and prevent the suffering of countless others who would come after her with similar stories. I'm grateful that Alex's mom credited me for her daughter's peace and purpose in the last months of her life, but Alex is the true hero. She found ways to impact others that transcended her death.

In many ways, Alex and I are not so different; it's just that I have been given more days to complete my mission. From the time I was young, I have been searching for answers, for truth and meaning—one part science and another part faith. In today's polarized world, my commitment to the divine and to scientific rigor may seem contradictory, but I believe this union is where true transformation of the human spirit has always been found. The type of medicine I now practice is incredibly complex, measuring and correcting individual biochemical imbalances through lab testing and careful application of supplements and medications along with prescribing dietary and lifestyle changes. But every instance of healing I've witnessed can be distilled down to a far simpler transformation: Believing something else is possible; embracing hope. This is how we become open to the unexpected. When we have clear goals, a pathway to reach them, and the belief in our ability to follow that path we are able to embrace hope. This is the first step to healing.

No matter who you are, life will always bring challenges, each of which provides an opportunity to either give up or build more resilience. Whether you are personally struggling with illness or some other challenge in life, I assure you that this book is meant for you. This is my own story of climbing life's mountains and striving for the inspired view, no matter how difficult it may be. Based on the inspiration Alex found to live life fully in her last months and her mom's description of her final smile, the view from the top is breathtaking.

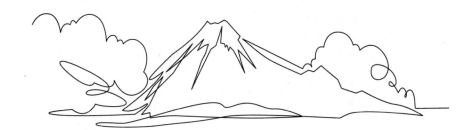

CHAPTER 1

Step Outside the Lines

I've always thought a mountain is a magnificent metaphor for life. From a distance the ascent looks clear and smooth, but once you actually set out for the summit you discover precarious valleys and ridges along the way. If your internal compass isn't set to keep climbing, every stumble will give you an excuse to turn back.

—OPRAH WINFREY

MAGICAL RED SLIPPERS

A SINGLE CRISP OCTOBER DAY CHANGED MY LIFE FOREVER. I'M QUITE
sure if I'd had any sense at all I would have suggested a smaller objective
than the thousand-foot-tall Third Flatiron—the largest and most iconic
of colossal rock formations that tower over Boulder, Colorado—for my
first climb. I had no idea what I was getting into, but I think that's the
beauty of it. We rarely go into a life-changing experience understanding
how much we will be transformed in the process. More often, we wake
up under ordinary circumstances, just as I did that day, hearing the
alarm clock beeping loudly, pulling me out of a delicous slumber. This
challenge had begun at a coffee shop about two months prior when I
was telling my friend Topher about some of my life's hardest lessons.
He paused and looked at me with a twinkle in his eye and blurted out,
"Would you like to go rock climbing?"

Never one to shy away from the hint of a new adventure, I exuber-
antly agreed, and we picked an autumn day for the climb. Facing my
fears and overcoming challenges had always delivered valuable lessons
in the past. Topher, an expert rock climber, promised to provide all
the equipment I would need, except climbing shoes. While I had
absolutely zero experience climbing, I believed that I could accom-
plish whatever I put my mind to. I also knew I was perfectly capable
of finding the perfect pair of shoes for any occasion, including rock
climbing.

On the day prior to our climb, just off the set of a televised interview and still dressed in a bright blue Calvin Klein sleeveless sheath
and patent leather four-inch heels, I walked confidently into REI. The
salesclerk gave my friend, Ilene Naomi, and me a once-over, paused
awkwardly, most likely wondering if I had accidently walked into the
wrong store, and asked, "May I help you?"

I giggled and said, "Yes, I need a pair of climbing shoes! I've never
climbed before, but I am going to climb the Flatirons tomorrow. Can
you help me?"

My friend and I proceeded to laugh hysterically at the antics of trying on rock climbing shoes in a dress more appropriate for Michigan Avenue than Pearl Street, jokingly asking which style and color went best with my dress. I settled on a darling bright red pair that stood out among the other options. They reminded me of the slippers worn by Dorothy in *The Wizard of Oz*, which would magically transport her to another time and place—not too far from the truth, considering what was in store for me the next day—so I immediately christened them my "magical red slippers."

The following morning at the base of the Empire State Building–sized rampart of weathered red sandstone, Topher pointed upward and said, "Here we are!" I was hit with the first twinges of fear, and the voice in my head said, "What the heck do you think you are doing?" I took a sip from my water bottle, steadied my heart rate with a slow, deep breath, and put on my magical red slippers.

POWER OF WISDOM

Topher gave me a brief lesson on the basics, summarizing a three-day climbing clinic in a little over ten minutes. He showed me how to angle my climbing shoes to match the angle of the rock where I wanted to stand, and I bravely took my very first step. I was climbing! I fooled gravity with my neophyte bravado—for about half a second. I slipped, skittering a short distance down the rock to land awkwardly on the forest floor, skinning my knuckles in the process. Licking the blood off my hand, I tried to shrug off the inauspicious start, but it did cross my mind that if I couldn't climb the first six inches without falling off, it didn't bode well for the next thousand feet.

Topher next explained that I would belay (pass the rope through a friction device and hold him if he fell) as he would lead a pitch (a section of the climb), placing safety equipment in cracks in the rock along the way to protect him if he fell. When he reached the end of the rope, he would stop at an anchor point and our roles would switch. Now he would belay me while I climbed. I would be responsible for removing the safety equipment, which is ingeniously designed to hold strong under the force of a fall but also be removed easily.

I was reminded of other times when trust was absolute. Trust is a part of the fabric of life, for good or bad. I'd trusted men who betrayed me and surgeons who saved me, but I knew that nothing in life could be accomplished without trust. Topher was a forty-year rock climbing veteran who started guiding climbers at fourteen years old under the tutelage of his mountain guide father. My life would be in his hands, and his in mine. If he trusted me, surely I could trust him.

There was a deep wisdom in my decision to be there that day—the kind of wisdom born of equal parts science and faith. This wisdom had been behind virtually every challenge I'd overcome in my life. As we geared up at the bottom of the mountain, I felt both aspects strongly. Science told me that by climbing with an experienced guide, I'd be safer than I had been driving the ten miles from my home to the base of the mountain that morning. I had faith in a higher power to protect me and also in my own ability to face new challenges and figure things out. I believed strongly that the answers would always come as I needed them.

Science gives us the information we need to make decisions. Faith gives us the confidence to act on those decisions while facing the inevitable uncertainty that is always present. Science and faith combine with experience, the most powerful (and often painful) teacher in my life, to form wisdom. On this day, wisdom is what drove me to believe there was a powerful lesson ahead in this brand-new experience.

EMBRACING FEAR

We tied into the rope, and I settled into my first belay. To distract my mind from the taste of my own blood, I wrapped both my hands around the rope confidently, partly because that's what I was told to do and partly because it gave me a tactile sense of absolute trust in the process, something to hold on to.

By the time Topher stopped to belay me, he was a tiny figure outlined against the periwinkle sky far above. I reached out and touched the jagged rock face, wondering how I could ever climb it. The surface wasn't like a ladder but rather a rippled, smooth wall with nothing more than small edges and pockets scattered randomly across its surface. I looked up from where my fingertips touched the stone just a few feet above the ground, pointing toward a thousand feet of rock rising above, and whispered to myself, "How in the world?"

My mind soon became laser focused as I took my time finding the next place to put the toe of my new climbing shoe. I felt equal parts excitement and terror. I could hear my own heart beating as I deliberately inhaled slowly and began to discover a new rhythm. I was reminded of looking up the one hudred-twenty-foot-tall grain leg on our family farm when I was only eight or nine years old as my brothers dared me to climb to the top. Before long, I found myself on top with a bird's-eye view of the surrounding farmland, trying to prove to my brothers that I was strong and brave, just like them. I remember the terrifying feeling as the wind blew through my hair, causing the tower to sway inches left and right and making me feel as if I were going to blow right off. I suppressed my fear and held on tight. Even then, long before I had studied the physiology of breathing, I realized that by focusing on controlling my breath, I could also control my anxiety and fear.

But it turns out that even though suppressing unsettling emotions might have been a good coping mechanism when I was young, over time it does more harm than good. As I started up the steep rock face, I did my best to let fear pulse through me in a natural rhythm.

> Being brave is not the absence of
> fear but allowing yourself to feel the
> fear and choosing to do it anyway.

At first, I was unsure in my movements, leaning too close to the rock and using far too much energy, but after the first few tentative steps I began to have a pleasant realization: *I knew this dance.* Rock climbing melded perfectly with my past in so many ways. To climb a mountain takes faith, and ever since I was a little girl, faith made me brave and allowed me to believe I could do anything I put my mind to. Faith gave me hope, a beam of light piercing through the darkness of fear.

This might have been my first climb, but I had been practicing this dance for as long as I could recall: the dance of transforming fear into hope; the dance of trusting the process; the dance where faith is the perfect partner, no matter what music is playing; the dance of embracing the fullness of life and moving to my soul's unique music while engaging my body and mind in the process of forward movement, engaging in the healing power of play and creativity. I was dancing!

When I reached Topher's airy perch at the top of the first pitch, he tied me into an anchor he'd set in the rock and congratulated me on my first rock climbing experience. Then he proceeded to explain that now we could still turn back, but once we went up higher, going back down would be difficult.

This implicit challenge only added to my sense of adventure as tendrils of fear enveloped my psyche. He was warning me that soon we would be committed and there would be no turning back. What he didn't know was that I was no stranger to a challenge.

In fact, the sense of challenge boosted my motivation. There was nothing he could have said that would have motivated me more to continue upward. Just tell me I can't do something, and I'll prove you wrong!

Some sensations were new—jagged edges of rock digging into my fingertips and the weight of my entire body balancing on a single toe, perilous but at the same time bizarrely reassuring. But other feelings were familiar, like the acrid smell of my own adrenaline-induced perspiration and the sensation of my heart pumping what seemed like a million beats per minute.

> A quiet feeling of pride came with believing in myself, acting with assured conviction, and trusting that it would all work out—the dance of faith over fear to my soul's unique song. I had done this before!

EXPERIENCING FLOW

My world simplified into the binary of stone and sky, with the forest and city far below. With commitment in charge, fear soon gave way to a brilliantly exhilarating high of norepinephrine and dopamine—the natural chemicals our body produces to help inspire us to do impossible things. I had no choice but to stay present, not looking back or too far ahead. As I hung precariously on the side of the mountain hundreds of feet above the ground, I realized that if I looked down, my fear would overpower my courage. I chose to deliberately minimize looking down so that I could focus on just the rock beneath me. Peering upward at the entirety of the climb that rose above was likewise overwhelming. The only moment that mattered was *now*.

While resting on the airy belay ledges better suited for eagles than humans, I let my mind wander. I was reminded of other watershed moments in my life: my first kiss, the admissions interview at Loyola medical school, a shocking phone call from my doctor informing me of a life-threatening diagnosis, holding my grandfather's hand as he took his last breath, and cradling in my arms the newborn baby of a patient who had been told she could never have children. Some of these moments I count among the best moments of my life, and others the worst, but all of them deserve equal credit for shaping the person I am today. This glorious mountain was about to join that list.

These milestones in my life all shared something in common, something that has long been associated with activities like rock climbing or sports performance but has been left out of healing discussions: *flow*. Flow is that seamless merging of the past and present into absolute immersion in the moment. The performance element of flow is well understood, while its therapeutic healing potential has received less attention, which is unfortunate because experiencing flow is a medicine available to everyone. Experiencing flow is powerful; it's a heady drug! I'd felt it every day in my clinic while listening to patients tell me their story and helping them find solutions to their health problems. I felt it when I was deep in research, seeking answers to my own health issues and those of my patients. And I felt it hiking in the mountains of Colorado, writing a new blog article, playing fetch with my puppy, or listening to classical music. Now I was feeling it on the side of a cliff half a mile above the rooftops of my home.

I kept the words of Glennon Doyle, author of *Untamed*, in my mind: "We can do hard things!" As I clung to the rock, I was filled with conflicting emotions: terror from the ever-growing void beneath my feet and an absolute faith in my ability to see things through. When the climb became more difficult, I began to sing hymns softly to myself, not caring if the other climbers heard me.

Climbing also forced me to take advantage of opportunities to rest, which is not my strong suit. On the farm, resting was seen as nonproductive, and I had rarely rested in medical school or in my first years as a practicing physician unless I was bedridden. As we approached the summit, the natural adrenaline high began to wane, my legs felt like jelly, and I noticed my hands shaking as I grabbed the next hold. When I got to the last step, I reached up to grasp the last fin of this ancient rock and felt such a surge of emotion that I started softly crying. I can hardly explain the relief and pride that filled my heart at that moment.

I sat on top with one leg hanging over the thousand-foot face we'd just climbed and the other over the backside of the rock formation. Looking down at what I'd just done, my mind could not wrap itself around the magnitude of it all. It was the first time all day that I was able to look down and appreciate the mountain as an ally, a source of motivation rather than an adversary. The very thing I had been afraid of was now giving me exhilarating joy and power. It was another strangely familiar feeling. I felt like a queen at the top of that mountain—not the traditional version of a monarch with unyielding power but my own newly empowered version, believing in my ability to overcome any obstacle, embracing my purpose and meaning in life, and showing up without apology.

Part of it was the feeling that inspires so many people to pursue adrenaline-fueled adventure sports and creative pursuits. The exhilarating high found in flow is certainly a factor, but there is far more to it than just a neurobiological chemical rush. For me, rock climbing exemplified every challenge I'd faced in my life—the dance that transforms the impossible into the possible and finally into something tangible, a priceless memory that would bolster me through the next challenge.

I sat there, still shaking a little, and whispered, "Thank you." My heart was filled with gratitude. Despite having been ravaged by deadly diseases, I was still strong and resilient. Despite challenges, or maybe because of them, life had been more rewarding than I'd ever imagined. I looked over at Topher and with tears in my eyes said, "Thank you. Thank you for inviting me on this adventure. Thank you for believing I had the courage and strength even when I hardly trusted myself. Thank you for creating safety for me along the way."

It was only after we were back on the ground that he told me, "Jill, in all my forty years of rock climbing, I have never taken anyone there for their first climb." He had noticed something different in me, a resilience that I wasn't even consciously aware of myself.

Many of us go out of our way to travel to exotic locations or take part in dangerous new adventures, like rock climbing, that force us to step outside our comfort zone and address our fears head-on or learn new skills. But why? Because it brings out the best in us! We find strength and resilience that we didn't even realize we had!

What if you could do this with your own life, your own challenges, your own physical suffering or emotional trauma? What if every day of life became an adventure, an opportunity to grow as a result of choosing to face challenges of all types—chosen adventures, like climbing, but also daily, unexpected happenings that we didn't choose?

> What if we let the everyday, unexpected
> events become our rock climbing
> adventures, explicit challenges
> to see what we are made of?

My first rock climbing experience reminded me of how life's adventures often hide unexpected lessons (or unexpected miracles), revealing to us a deep inner strength that we didn't know we possessed. Not long after, I found an equally valuable unexpected miracle by picking up a simple box of colored pencils and a piece of paper.

COLORING OUTSIDE THE LINES

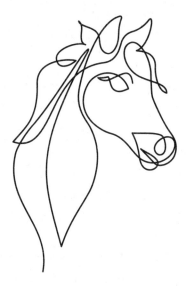

The farm where I grew up contained a beautiful but harsh reality: we had everything we needed to survive but could easily lose it all at any time. My dad, Ken, mortgaged the farm each year to purchase seed and equipment, a gamble on the crops yielding enough to pay off the debt. Mine was a childhood of practicality, arduous work, and faith that God would provide each year. I had never experienced a dream-like world of pink princess dresses or unicorns. My parents didn't even allow us to believe in Santa Claus. My make-believe consisted of tree houses and sand cakes, practical things mimicking real-life lessons.

Yet in my heart I cherished the idea that there was more to life than the practical dirt under my feet. I was often chastised for daydreaming instead of finishing my chores, and I'd get lost for hours in my own personal make-believe reality. Now, decades later, with the very same creative energy of my childhood that I had disregarded as being "impractical," I picked up my colored pencils and a piece of paper and began coloring. I was drawn to color mythical creatures, magical unicorns. It opened my awareness to the beautiful opportunity for my own transformation through curiosity and creativity. The act of embracing my imagination and play was every bit as enlightening as the rock climb and allowed me to realize that my inner child had a lesson or two to teach me.

According to medieval myths, the unicorn is a wild creature that could purify water or cure the sick with a touch of its horn. This creature was said to see into the heart of any situation and true character of any person. While drawing, I realized that I was related to this lovely mythical creature. I wanted to help my patients see their amazing potential and encourage them to ponder limitless possibilities even during times when pain and discouragement clouded their own vision.

Our bodies are born with the innate intelligence and design to heal. Anyone who has ever cut themselves has seen the incredible transformation of the skin as it changes over a matter of few days from an angry, broken wound to pristine skin. We each possess an intrinsic intelligence that can transform suffering into triumph, weakness into strength, and trauma into empowerment. This unconscious wisdom is knowing what needs to change and trusting in our body's natural ability to carry it out. Like the unicorn, this healing wisdom is already within each of us.

So how do we tap into these natural healing abilities, our instinctive heart-based knowing and childlike curiosity? In a word: *intuition*. For the majority of my life, I trusted my analytical mind to figure things out, but this carried me only so far. I eventually learned that there is a great deal of incoming information and processing that takes place outside our conscious awareness but that lends great value to our decision-making. Part of gaining wisdom is accumulating a lifetime of experience, which supplies clues to fund our pattern-recognition system with thousands of data points that we rely on to make the next decision. Intuition becomes more valuable when its foundation is life experience, which also means the older we are, the more powerful it becomes as our guide. Intuition leads us to try things we would never have dreamed possible if we had remained tethered to a purely analytical view of the world. This is how I have come to experience unexpected miracles—whether it be through climbing or coloring or introducing new treatment protocols to my patients. Each of these pursuits inspired me to embrace a different dimension of myself than I was used to. Trying something totally different, outside our comfort zone, outside the lines, allows us to view life circumstances in a different light and see fresh, unique solutions that move us toward healing.

> I used to let fear of judgment keep me
> from vulnerability, hiding the parts
> of myself I was ashamed of, those I
> had deemed unworthy or unlovable.

According to Daniel Kahneman, professor emeritus at Princeton University's School of Public and International Affairs and author of *Thinking, Fast and Slow*, there have long been two systems that our brain uses to solve problems. System 1 is fast, automatic, frequent, emotional, and relatively unconscious. System 2 is slow, effortful, logical, calculating, and conscious. While I had long used System 2 to get through my training and practice medicine effectively, I was now learning the magnificent power of System 1 to reach a new level of healing and teaching my patients do the same.

Harnessing the healing power of intuition begins by trusting and accepting yourself completely, even the parts that you may feel are less worthy of love and acceptance. If you are not sure what intuition feels like, close your eyes and imagine the purest, loveliest, truest part of yourself whispering in your ear. Brené Brown speaks of this level of authenticity in her book *Daring Greatly*: "We cultivate love when we allow our most vulnerable and powerful selves to be deeply seen and known, and when we honor the spiritual connection that grows from that offering with trust, respect, kindness and affection."[1]

But what if throwing away the idea that we need to be perfect leaves more room for joy and authenticity? What if it is possible to overcome our challenges in ways that are easier than we ever dreamed possible, filled with exciting, adventure-filled twists and turns and unexpected miracles along the way?

What wild or unconventional voice is calling *you*? Can you hear it? It might rattle the old vision you have of yourself and your former beliefs about your world, daring you to become more authentic, more open to where life is leading you, and more willing to surrender and let go of control, even to do something you never dreamed of, like going rock climbing.

> **Listen! That voice is calling you to be true to yourself.**

Love all the parts of yourself that used to live in the shadows. You might find, like I did, that some of the most challenging circumstances turn out to be great catalysts for profound growth and awakening. What follows is how it happened for me, but I tell it only so that you might see your own story, like a reflection on the surface of a still pond, be encouraged, and know that it can happen for you too! This is the path to finding resiliency and unexpected miracles and living a life of joy and vibrancy.

What Is Functional Medicine?

Functional medicine is built on the foundation of trust rooted in the patient–practitioner partnership—a unique, deeply connected relationship that, at its core, ensures the greatest progression and expression of individual health for all people.

It is a systems-based, biology-based model that empowers patients and practitioners to work together to achieve the highest expression of health by addressing the underlying causes of disease. It utilizes personalized therapeutic interventions to support individuals in achieving optimal wellness.

The Institute of Functional Medicine describes it in the following way:

> The functional medicine model is an individualized, patient-centered, science-based approach that empowers patients and practitioners to work together to address the underlying causes of disease and promote optimal wellness. It requires a detailed understanding of each patient's genetic, biochemical, and lifestyle factors and leverages that data to direct personalized treatment plans that lead to improved patient outcomes.

> By addressing root cause, rather than symptoms, practitioners become oriented to identifying the complexity of disease. They may find one condition has many different causes and, likewise, one cause may result in many different conditions. As a result, functional medicine treatment targets the specific manifestations of disease in everyone.[2]

Learn more at www.ReadUnexpected.com/Resources.

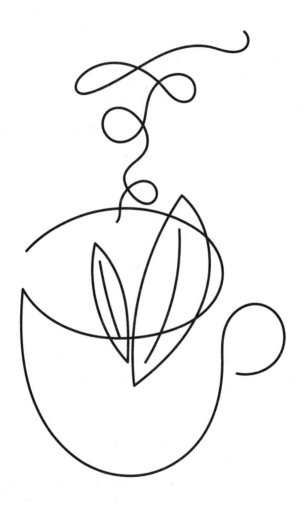

CHAPTER 2

Trust Your Intuition

*Be who God made you to be and
you will set the world on fire.*
—St. Catherine of Siena

WALKING THE BEANS

EVERY ONCE IN A WHILE, WHEN I AM HOLDING A STETHOSCOPE TO A patient's chest listening to their heart, I find myself looking at my own hands. I used to be embarrassed of my large, strong hands, but I'm not anymore. I see the visible vasculature, toned muscles, strong knuckles, and scarred skin shaped by a life far removed from the clinical environment of my functional medicine practice, and I'm reminded of the long-ago moments that shaped these hands. The ice-cold water running over them on cool fall days as my brothers, sister, and I picked, washed, and quartered apples for the cider press, and the painful pleasure of warmth returning to my fingers as I held them next to the space heater set up in the steel Quonset that also housed many of the farm implements. My dad's own muscular forearms and hands—legendary across the farmlands of Woodford County, Illinois, for looking more like those of a professional athlete than a farmer—would twist the crank on the cider press, and precious gold liquid would run from between the wooden slats and into a vat below. The reward for our demanding work was that first sip of fresh, golden apple cider. Drinking the nectar from fruit that had been just hours before hanging in our orchard and connected to the earth's nutrients and the sun's energy, and feeling it pass into the inner world of my body, made all the effort worthwhile. Tasting the sweet, crispy tartness of a glass of apple cider still brings back nostalgia of a simpler time in my childhood where I witnessed the wonder of a bountiful harvest, learned the importance of hard work in overcoming challenges, and experienced the inevitable rewards that followed.

Long before I ever strapped on a blood pressure cuff or listened to the intimate rhythms of a heartbeat through a stethoscope, I was a farm girl. My childhood home was a simple, two-story white farmhouse with a shaded front porch surrounded by a copse of trees to protect us from the wind. Nurturing life was our daily goal—either our own or that of our crops. We spent countless hours at the red picnic table on the front porch, shucking sweet corn to freeze, stemming straw-berries, or shelling peas from our half-acre garden. Sometimes we'd have our extended family over, cousins and all, for a "corn-shucking party" or to help with the cider-making. My great-great-grandfather Hodel and his two brothers emigrated from Germany in the 1870s and purchased a small farm in central Illinois near the small town of Roanoke. The three were as prolific with procreation as they were with farming, so when the Hodel family would get together, we could move mountains due to sheer numbers.

In the late summer, my paternal grandmother, Margaret, also known as "Sparky," who never had a single snow-white hair out of place, would take orders for fruits and vegetables that we didn't grow ourselves, and my ornery grandfather, Glen, would drive his rusty, hunter green, two-ton truck up to Michigan to bring back a load of fresh blueberries, Bing cherries, peaches, and other seasonal fruit. He would put an ad in the local newspaper announcing his plan, and neighbors would come from everywhere to visit Grandpa Glen's farm, located no more than a mile, as the crow flies, from our farmstead to pick up their orders. We'd stop by to help unload and sort the produce, and he'd have a prank ready for us, like a stick of gum that would disappear into his fist as soon as we'd reach for it, our feigned disappointment matched by his mischievous, round-faced grin, eyes sparkling from behind horn-rimmed glasses. Back home, we'd help my mother, Kathy, prepare the fruit and vegetables to be stored in two huge chest freezers in our dusty, dirt-floored basement pantry. Every year we worked hard to store enough food to last our family of seven through the long, gray Illinois winter.

Our farmhouse was dwarfed by four on-site silver grain bins and a tall grain leg rising more than one hundred twenty feet in the center. It became a terrifying adventure on that hot summer day when I climbed up to the top on a dare from my older brother, Jeff. I remember my heart pounding as I looked straight ahead, refusing to look down as I clung to the cold metal rungs, which rose like a ladder into the Illinois sky. The scary climb was worth it just for the view of our farm from above with our house; garden; outbuildings for storing machines, chemicals, and tools; and a school bus–sized tank for diesel fuel all clustered together. Beyond the house and farm infrastructure, fields of soybeans and corn stretched as far as the eye could see on the horizon.

Although I wouldn't have been able to put it into words at the time, intuitively I had a feeling that the sea of life that I gazed on from my bird's-eye perch was not only nourishing my body and my family but also slowly poisoning me. On the surface, I lived in one of the healthiest environments on earth, but in stark contrast with my wholesome, Norman Rockwellesque world of love, faith, and nurturing life, the farm was assaulting my body's unique biochemistry, starting before I was born. As my mom says now, after praying me through too many deadly illnesses, "We lived around the enemy."

Genetically modified plants that could produce their own insecticide or resist glyphosate toxicity while the weeds around them died had yet to be invented, so one of our jobs as children was to "walk the beans" and pull weeds from between the rows of soybeans. In one of our family photos, the whole family is walking the beans, and most of the family appears happy and cheerful as they walk along the rows. Not me. I am rubbing a fist in red, swollen eyes, nose scrunched up ready to sneeze, rashes breaking out all over my body, looking miserable and overwhelmed. Upon returning to the house after walking the beans, I would sneeze endlessly and then fall into an exhausted sleep for hours while my brothers and little sister played outside.

Many of my earliest memories are colored by my severe allergies, which made my days of working anywhere near fields pure torture. Looking back, I realize that turning to intellectual pursuits instead of physical labor was my first attempt at shaping my environment for my own health. I fell in love with books because they offered me an alternative reality and kept me out of the fields and away from the corn and soybean dust that was so toxic to my system.

I intuitively came to understand that farm girls don't cry or complain. While this created a foundation of resiliency and fortitude, it also caused me emotional damage as I tried my best to suppress my delicate, sensitive nature. In a fifth-grade school project I wrote in carefully crafted block letters, "I would feel more important to my dad if I didn't have so many allergies so I could help him more." As a tough farmer, my father, Ken, didn't share his troubles openly when I was young. I followed my daddy's lead and tried my best to suffer quietly too. It wasn't until later in life that I learned suppressing our emotions is toxic for the body and soul. This was something passed down in my stoic German family for many generations and was especially evident in my grandmother, Margaret, who lived her entire life in quiet surrender, working hard to raise her family but suffering from depression throughout her last decade of life, never having spoken of the hardships of being in a verbally abusive marriage while raising five children. My mother, Kathy, had a brighter outlook on the world, a perspective to which I owe my own optimism, but she rarely sat down to rest and never complained either. It was not a shock when my maternal grandmother told me her mother had been the same, and I realized this pattern of not allowing ourselves to rest, of suffering silently, and of being driven by the teaching that "idleness is a sin" was a recipe deeply ingrained in my family for many generations.

I carried a great deal of guilt about my allergies, subconsciously feeling I was less worthy of love or acceptance due to my inability to do manual labor like the boys, who pulled more weight than I did because they could work hard all day outside. It was an unfair shame (as most shame is) because, as part of a family with five children, there was plenty of work left to be done inside the house, and I spent most days cooking, cleaning, and taking care of my younger siblings.

Modeling Healthy Behavior for Our Children

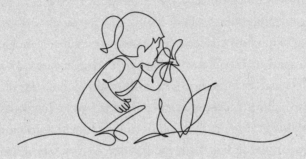

We have all heard the flight attendant's instructions to put on your own oxygen mask before that of your children. Children learn by our example, so modeling healthy self-care is the perfect way to begin nurturing your children's health.

Here's a quick quiz to see how you are doing:

- Do you exercise or move your body at least thirty minutes every day?
- Are you choosing to model healthy dietary habits, avoiding processed foods? One of the easiest ways to get started is to cut out all processed sugar.
- Do you make quiet time for prayer or meditation before you start your day?
- Do you average at least seven hours of sleep each night?
- Are you allowing yourself to express a full range of emotions, including sadness or anger, giving your children permission to do the same without judgment?
- Do you maintain a healthy balance between work and play and encourage your children to do the same?
- Are you choosing to practice nonjudgmental language and open communication with your partner, modeling kindness and curiosity and listening to understand?

ROLLIE'S COUNTRY KITCHEN

The pressure I felt to participate alongside my brothers and father in the farm work was entirely of my own creation. I so desperately wanted to be able to join them, and sometimes I was willing to pay the price to be one of the boys. Partly I wanted to contribute and partly I adored the trivial things, like climbing into my dad's truck for a trip into town for breakfast and coffee at Rollie's.

The 1970s coffee shop in Roanoke, Illinois, bore little resemblance to a 2020s coffee shop in Boulder, Colorado, where my medical practice is now—at Rollie's Country Kitchen, nobody was in a hurry, and a bottomless cup of coffee with a farmer-sized serving of hash browns, bacon, and eggs cost less than a cappuccino with a dusting of cinnamon in Boulder. Maybe this is why, to this day, coffee shops are my happy place. I think this feeling goes back to when my dad would invite one of us to join him for a trip into town to get breakfast (and hear the latest farmer gossip) at Rollie's. Joining Dad was a great source of joy, and my siblings and I loved the opportunity to be his sidekick for the morning. He made sure to take each of us in turn, and our excitement at being the one to go with him never faded.

But no matter the inexpensive grub, going to Rollie's was pricey for me. My dad's truck was always full of corn and soybean dust, layered so thick that we could sign our names in it on the dashboard. The moment I climbed into the truck, I would start sneezing, and I'd continue throughout the trip, arriving back home with my eyes swollen and my energy sapped. My mom would give me a dose of Benadryl to soothe the allergic response, and I'd retreat to my room and sleep for hours. I realize now that I spent a good part of my life on the farm vacillating between two extremes. Part of the time I thought, *I'm tough! I can do this!* But most of the time I thought, *What is wrong with me? Why can't I keep up with the others?*

My siblings and I were taught to support each other and be kind, to find joy in the process, and most of all to have faith that all things work out in the end. Demanding work without complaint, self-reliance, and the discipline of healthy habits was a way of life, as was seeking deeper knowledge and the high value of lifelong learning and education. We were free to argue and debate during dinner, but before we were excused from the table, my parents insisted that we memorize educational quotes or verses of Scripture. On Sunday after church, we'd gather in our seventies-style living room, which was decorated with dark wood paneling, red-and-black velvet wall coverings, and wooden railroad ties crossing the ceiling at regular intervals, and listen attentively while my father would read to us, usually a hero's story like one about Corrie ten Boom, Anne Frank, or Brother Andrew—a real adult chapter book! What I thought was a tragedy as a child (not being allowed to watch television) became one of my parents' greatest gifts by inspiring us to find more creative pursuits, such as making tree houses, selling lemonade by the roadside, or filling my mother's kitchen with an assortment of arts and crafts. I cherished wintertime when the crops were dormant, allergy symptoms were minimal, and workdays were shorter. The long evenings were spent playing board games, having competitive ping-pong tournaments, or taking part in some other creative family entertainment, including the occasional old-fashioned neighborhood taffy pull. Sometimes my dad would even take the television out of the closet for family movie night, complete with homemade caramel corn and sliced apples from our orchard.

Fresh, homegrown food made up much of our diet, and the memory of plucking fresh strawberries and harvesting red raspberries or peas from the vines and popping them into my mouth still makes me grin. I had a rule that for every berry or pea that I put in my basket, I got to eat one. I would go home without much of an appetite, my mother slightly suspicious as to my meager harvest and the obvious stains on my lips. I am sure she guessed why I wasn't hungry for lunch. Another one of my jobs was to use our bright blue

Dixon Zero Turn riding lawn mower to mow the nearly two acres of grass that surrounded the farmstead and house. I loved the time in the sunshine, driving that lawn mower to create beautiful, manicured lines on the diagonal and listening to popular 80s music on my Walkman, but I paid dearly for it with fatigue from the allergies that put me to sleep within a few hours of completing the task. We had clean air, plenty of physical exercise, and a large garden filled with organic, homegrown produce, but something about this land where I grew up was contributing to my symptoms of severe allergies, eczema, and fatigue as a child.

I was frequently charged with watching my younger siblings, and as anyone who has lived on a farm knows, there are dangers lurking everywhere. The combination of responsibility and the inherent dangers on the farm combined to form some of the most stressful memories of my life. I will never forget one time I let my youngest brother swing on the hose that hung from the gasoline tank in the yard. Without warning, the hose suddenly detached from the tank, showering my little brother in gasoline. I was frozen in horror for a brief second, not knowing what to do, before I came to my senses and grabbed him out from under the flow and ran into the house frantically yelling for someone to come help me shut off the tank. Shortly after, John, a driver who was there to pour concrete for a project, unconsciously lit up a cigarette, nearly throwing the match onto the gravel where the thousands of gallons of fuel had just moments before spilled. My mother came flying out of the house frantically trying to catch his attention before he caused a massive explosion. That might have ended my story right there, but fortunately she stopped him before he threw down the match.

Life on the farm was also the beginning of my medical education. It is where I learned to trust my intuition even if I couldn't explain or understand it. It is also where I learned to respect the world of science as well as the overarching value of faith—the two driving forces in my own survival and the miracles I witness each day. It's not a stretch to speculate that, were it not for my exquisite sensitivities, I might be a farmer instead of a doctor; the two are not so far apart. While I gravitated toward functional medicine, seeking the root cause of disease, my older brother, Jeff, has become a progressive innovator in farming, committing his life to delving into the root cause of crop success and failure in a quest to sustain the healthiest soils for the highest-quality crops. When we get together, we often talk about how similar the microbiome of the body and the biome of the soil really are and how they're also inseparable: the health of the microbiome and gut are very related to the soil quality where our food is grown. Soil is a living, breathing ecosystem and perhaps one of the most complex structures known to man. As we continue to alter our fertile soils with the application of chemicals, herbicides, and pesticides, destroying the organisms within or altering the rich top layer, we unwittingly change the nutrient content and microsystem that supports this critical component of the world's food system.

> I used to say disease begins in the gut,
> but now I often go a step further and
> say disease really begins in our soils.

BUCKET FULL OF TOXINS

The rich, dark soils surrounding my family's farm not only provided for our way of life and sustenance but were also the breadbasket of the world. By the time I was born in 1976, a single farmer was providing enough food to feed eighty people, aided by the invention of twenty-foot-wide tiling disks, herbicide applicators that could spray sixteen rows of crops in a single pass, and advances in chemicals that transformed farming as much as any invention since the plow. My father did the same thing all the farmers around us did. He sprayed insecticide on the crops to keep the bugs off and then herbicide to kill the weeds during planting season. We were the guinea pigs of agricultural chemical use. There has been some regulation since then but not enough to keep babies from taking their very first breath with hundreds of toxins already in their systems (based on a 2005 study showing an average of two hundred chemicals in the umbilical cord blood of newborns, including pesticides and components of coal, gasoline, and garbage[3]).

My mother handled her other four pregnancies with ease, but her pregnancy with me was the most difficult. She suffered from heartburn, sleepless nights, allergies, and sinus infections, and when she traveled to the city, she found the car fumes were intolerable. When I came home from the hospital with a staph infection in my belly button and a prescription for antibacterial cream to treat it, she was shocked. How could a baby born from the perfect environment of the womb develop an infection?

That was just the beginning. Two years later my tonsils grew so swollen that I couldn't swallow, and, after my first round of oral antibiotics, they were surgically removed. By the time I was ten years old, I had taken nine rounds of antibiotics. All the other kids got chicken pox, but I got impetigo (infected crusts and scabs) on top of my chicken pox. I had pneumonia, multiple episodes of strep throat, and croup, scaring my parents by coughing like a barking seal in the middle of the night. I caught every cold that came by and took nine different medicines to help with eczema, itchy eyes, stuffy nose, and sneezing. Sometimes the rashes were so bad that I'd wake up in the morning and the sheets would be bloody from where I'd scratched my legs to the point of hemorrhage.

I didn't consider why I was suffering at the time, and I certainly didn't think the same farm that provided my family with nourishment might be poisoning my body, but intuitively I could feel that something was clearly different about my immune system. My mom always said that I was sensitive like a canary in a coal mine. When I was ten years old, she had her first epiphany, during a trip to the "big city" of Wisconsin Dells and our stay in a new hotel, that my issues somehow stemmed from the environment where we lived. In the hotel environment with air conditioner–filtered air, a pool adding humidity, and a clean, modern building free of mold and dust, I wasn't sneezy or itchy and had a surprising amount of energy.

I've learned that the best way to explain the body's capacity to handle toxins is to describe it like a bucket. If toxins are filling up the bucket at the same rate the body can rid itself of these toxins, the body continues to function fine. But if the toxins coming in exceed the bucket's capacity to hold them, they spill out over the top like water and we begin to have significant symptoms, resulting in conditions like inflammation, autoimmunity, allergies, or other chronic illnesses. We are genetically programmed with different-sized buckets or abilities to detoxify any incidental exposures. Unfortunately, I was born with a very small one. In time I learned that if I could reduce some of the toxic load and create more room or margin in the bucket, my body would do just fine.

> We don't need to eliminate all of the toxins, just enough to create space or margin in our bucket.

It turns out this concept of toxic load and teaching patients to reduce their exposures and toxic burden has become one of the core tenets of successful healing from complex chronic disease in my clinic.

PRAYER WARRIOR

My parents met on a blind double date with my Uncle John and Aunt Barb. My mother was only fourteen years old at the time, but my father immediately knew something was different about this girl.

What Things Contribute to Total Toxic Load?

Exotoxins

These are toxins that come from an outside source and fill our bucket:

- Heavy metals
- Solvents
- VOCs: volatile organic compounds
- Organophosphates
- Pesticides
- BPA: bisphenol A
- Phthalates
- Parabens
- EMFs: electromagnetic fields
- Heterocyclic amines
- Mold and mycotoxins
- POPs: persistent organic pollutants

Endotoxins

These are toxins that come from inside our bodies and fill our bucket:

- Intestinal bacteria (endotoxemia from lipopolysaccharides [LPS])
- Yeast/candida (which produce acetaldehyde)
- Toxins from other infections
- Food additives and chemical ingredients
- Food allergens
- Psychological stress
- Emotions like loneliness, anger, jealousy, or fear

Right away, her profound compassion and authenticity left an impression on him. Four years her senior, he went off to college shortly after they met but knew immediately in his heart that he wanted to marry this sensitive, faith-filled gal. So he waited four years until my mother turned eighteen. He proposed and they were married shortly after on August 30, 1970, in the presence of more than six hundred guests at the Apostolic Christian Church. A lively reception followed at my grandparents' home in Eureka, Illinois, on a day when the temperature reached nearly one hundred degrees. The church lacked air conditioning, and in the wedding photos, beads of sweat sparkle on the outside of my father's tie.

When my mother turned twenty years old, Dr. Riggert told her, "It would be a miracle if you were ever able to have children, Kathy." From age sixteen she had irregular menstrual cycles occurring only three or four times per year. After marrying my father, she went to nursing school and then to work for the local country doctor. Three years later, resigned to the fact that her deepest desire to have a large family would never happen, she began looking into fostering children. And as luck or faith would have it, within months she found out she was pregnant with the first of five children.

Farming was uncertain business in the 1980s, and my father recalls waking up at 3 a.m. one night with profound anxiety, knowing that if the crops didn't come in strong that year, the bank would take everything. He opened his worn, black King James Bible and read from Genesis 18:14: "Is anything too hard for the Lord?" He hand-wrote the verse on a piece of white cardboard in his classic lefty scrawl, and it remained framed in my parents' bedroom for the remainder of my childhood, a constant reminder that *nothing* is impossible. In these small ways, my parents contributed to my belief in miracles and that no dream or goal is too big, and in many ways they set me up for going places I never dreamed possible, like being the first woman (or man for that matter) in my family to become a doctor.

My precious mother is a prayer warrior and a saint. There is no doubt that the many hours she spent in prayer over me, wearing calluses on her knees, are part of the reason I feel God's nearness, protection, and provision in everything I do. I once heard that prayers on our behalf are like tears in a bottle that God collects. If that is the case, God must have a whole mansion full of bottles collecting my mother's prayers. The confidence I've felt, every single day of my life, that God will show up for me in miraculous ways was partially borne of a mother devoted to praying for her beloved family, consistently putting her needs aside, and demonstrating sacrifice, humility, and a servant heart and of a father who was steadfastly convinced that, with belief, anything is possible. Even if you don't believe the same way I do, it is a powerful healing tonic to embrace the belief that all our experiences have purpose and meaning, each one teaching us lessons and maturing our souls along this journey called life.

In hindsight, I can see how much my mother's faith helped her through her own challenges. She wanted nothing more than to raise a family, but her faith helped her accept that her one desire for children may never happen. I believe it afforded her a peaceful acceptance and contributed to her body's unexpected fertility and the miracle of a large family. I see this commonly in my clinical practice. The stress of trying hard to conceive often leads to frustration and sometimes failure to get pregnant despite trying everything. Then, as soon as the couple resigns themselves to the fact that they may not be able to conceive naturally, they unexpectedly find out they are pregnant.

Could my mother's own struggles with infertility, chronic fatigue, and migraine headaches have been evidence of her own body's toxic load accumulation, which may have been passed on to me in utero? We may never know for sure, but it is worth pondering for women wanting to conceive. It is advisable well before pregnancy to address toxic load to optimize your child's health. In any case, an understanding of all that my mother went through to give me life and her ongoing unconditional love and support has been an anchor and inspiration in each of the life challenges I have faced.

READING TROUBLE

IF MY MOM WERE IN ELEMENTARY SCHOOL TODAY, SHE WOULD BE diagnosed with dyslexia. She once told me about reading next to her classmate at a two-seater wooden desk. When her desk mate said, "Are you finished reading yet?" My mother felt ashamed of admitting that she was only a quarter way through, so she said, "Yes, I am." For the rest of her grade school education, she read only about half of the

Giving Babies a Clean Start

If you are trying to start a family or thinking about it, it's never too soon to consider how your choices will affect the health of your baby. Preconception tips focus on what you and your partner can do to ensure your best chance of having a healthy baby in the future.

Here are some of my top tips for preconception:
- Take a high-quality prenatal vitamin that includes methylated Bs and choline, along with omega-3 fatty acids (EPA and DHA).
- Stay active and maintain a healthy weight.
- Avoid smoking, drinking excessive alcohol, or consuming excessive stimulants like coffee.

- Clean up your diet. Avoid consuming foods with artificial hormones and pesticides. Avoid high-mercury fish and highly processed foods.
- Commit to clean air. Install a high-quality HEPA air filter with VOC filter in your home.
- Find a functional medicine doctor to assess your hormone levels, thyroid function, total toxic burden, overall gut health, and level of inflammation.
- Ask your doctor to check thyroid function if you have any risk factors.
- Detox your body at least six months prior to getting pregnant. If you don't have this time, it's best to focus on avoiding toxins versus working on aggressive detoxification. Toxins in a mother's body are passed to the baby through cord blood and breast milk.[4]

Thanks to Dr. Christine Maren for review.

books assigned because she was so slow. It wasn't until her pregnancy with me, at the age of twenty-four, that my dad encouraged her to pick up a book and start reading again.

"Kathy," he said, "it doesn't matter how slowly you go through the book; you can still learn to read." She took his words to heart, and during her difficult pregnancy with me she fell in love with reading for the first time in her life. She recently told me, "Jill, one of my greatest desires was that all of my children would develop a deep love and appreciation for reading." Was I, as a child in the womb, sensitive enough to feel and absorb my mother's newfound love of reading? Is it possible that my own love of reading began when my father gave my mother the courage to believe she was not stupid and could learn to read? I believe there is absolutely a connection.

Case in point, I recently came across new research that shed light on something my intuition has long suspected and I wish I would have known in my teens and twenties. I happen to belong to a category of people who are exquisitely sensitive to both the physical world and the emotional realm. In the minority, we are called Highly Sensitive Persons, or HSPs, a characteristic researched and discovered by Dr. Elaine Aron.

If you're not one, right now you're thinking, "Yeah right, that's not a real thing." If you're also an HSP, right now you're thinking, "I knew it! I knew there had to be more people out there like me!"

Whichever way you respond, Dr. Aron's insightful book *The Highly Sensitive Person* is a must-read—you'll never look at sensitivity or intuition the same. And if you ever partner with an HSP, you'll be nicely rewarded for your understanding!

This HSP characteristic is also called sensory processing sensitivity (SPS) and is recognized as a trait associated with greater responsiveness and sensitivity to stimuli. This is an inborn trait found in fifteen to twenty percent of the population, and it has also been identified in one hundred other species. I'm fairly sure my Havanese dog, Ravi, is an HSPooch. If I'm about to cry, he will whine to get up on my lap, ready and waiting to lick away the first tear. He mirrors my every mood and sometimes rests his head on my arm as I am writing and looks up at me with such curiosity and concern that I wonder if there is a human soul inside that sweet puppy heart of his. I love people and the energy of interactions with others, but I get easily overwhelmed and overstimulated by interaction, especially in large groups, and I need lots of alone time to think and to recharge my battery.

The HSP trait engenders a survival strategy that is a blessing and a curse. HSPs tend to be more observant, empathetic, emotionally responsive, and process the environment around them more deeply before acting. The downside is that we are also more easily overwhelmed; overstimulated by things that are too intense, like sound and light; and more susceptible to insidious environmental factors, like noxious smells or chemicals. This trait is often mistaken for shyness, cowardliness, and weakness, but the reality is that the HSP characteristic is an entirely unique way of perceiving the world. According to Dr. Aron, we HSPs benefit from an ability to process material at deeper levels, to learn without realizing we are learning, and to show an increased propensity for vigilance, concentration, accuracy, speed, and the detection of minor differences. The world might see us as lacking something others have, but we have superpowers hidden within our delicate constitutions. It is the gift of being overly sensitive that allows me to deeply tune in to my intuition and notice details in my patients' expressions and the way they answer certain questions that lead to the root cause of their problems and eventually the solution. As is so often the case, what at first glance is a problem turns out to be a superpower.

> The downside for HSPs is that our little teacup-sized toxin buckets overflow easily, so it is natural for us to define *toxin* as anything that decreases optimal vitality and function.

This hypersensitivity includes detection of chemical toxins, of course, but also the toxicity of stress, destructive relationships, and any stimulus that causes emotional or hormonal dysfunction. These wide-ranging toxins can damage anyone, but HSPs react to the toxicity at subclinical levels or doses lower than what would bother another person. As a result, most HSPs, over time, have become experts at reducing their toxic stress and environmental toxicity to a level that allows them to function. This means that, surprisingly, HSPs may be better prepared for life in our toxic world than others who are less sensitive.

Are You a Highly Sensitive Person?

1. Easily overwhelmed by things like bright lights, strong smells, coarse fabrics, or loud noises nearby?
2. Get rattled when you have a short amount of time to do a lot of different things?
3. Make a point of avoiding violent movies and TV shows?
4. Need to withdraw during busy days into bed or a darkened room where you can have privacy and relief from others?
5. Make it a high priority to avoid upsetting or over-whelming situations?
6. Notice delicate or fine scents, tastes, or sounds?
7. Have a rich and complex inner life?
8. Your parents or teachers saw you as a sensitive or gifted child

If you said yes to five or more of these, don't worry, you're normal. This trait is found in about 15 to 20 percent of the population.[5]

SENSITIVITY IS THE NEW SUPERPOWER

Environmental toxic load has increased so dramatically that researchers have given up on even being able to classify the increase, but estimates suggest a *few thousand* new chemicals are introduced into the environment each year.[6] However you count it, decades ago, our grandparents and great-grandparents did not grow up eating food laced with pesticides, breathing volatile organic compounds, or drinking water laced with pharmaceuticals, so their buckets could better accommodate their toxic load. On top of the chemical toxicity, those generations past didn't have an Internet to further overload them with the toxic stress of seeing the many tragic stories of famine, death, wars, or other calamities that make news around the world. What it means to be sensitive is changing.

Watching toxins wreak havoc on my own system, and on the lives of so many of my patients, and following the data that supports the HSP theory, I've become a firm believer that the HSP trait, toxic stress, and environmental illness are connected. These sensitivities are not only emotional; my HSP patients always have an increased physical sensitivity to toxic exposure as well. On the other side of the coin, my patients who are unusually sensitive also tend to be more willing to make necessary changes in their lives to improve their health.

Although I didn't understand I was an HSP when I was a kid, I did know that I often needed to retreat to recharge when life became overwhelming to my nervous system. Books were my sanctuary, an alternative universe, far from the place where the very air I breathed brought me to my knees. My parents were strong proponents of education and encouraged reading, but only after the work was done. I would often sneak away to my bedroom once my chores were done to read one of my beloved books. I cannot tell you the number of times I got into trouble for sneaking away to read. The message I got while I was very young was that rest is not okay and was punishable by a scolding. Imagine a child today getting in trouble for reading a book!

I still feel guilty when I sit down to enjoy a good book or try to rest without being productive. Somehow I got the subconscious message that I was worthy of love only when I was working or achieving something of significance. Savoring the stillness of a quiet morning has taken me my entire adult life to learn but has been at least as therapeutic as any medications or supplement. I have found that my intuition is always spot on, but it was so quiet in those early days when I didn't yet know how to listen to my heart. Although my sensitivity is a beautiful quality, I didn't always see it that way.

WHISPERS OF A HEALER

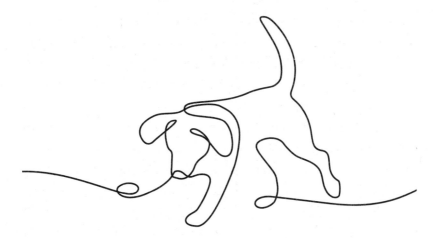

Many stray cats and dogs made our farm their home, but it was a dangerous place for animals and humans alike. It wasn't uncommon for a cat to limp onto the porch with a wound on her little paw or for a dog to get hit by a passing car. My earliest understanding that there was a healer inside me was when I saw the suffering of an animal or another human being.

My parents knew the farm environment was hard on animals, so they discouraged naming them and treating them like pets. But the lack of a name is no barrier to love. One of the stray dogs would run around the farm with me. I still have the image seared in my mind of seeing him run out into the road: hearing a car coming; trying to yell but my scream silent, my voice frozen in horror; then finding his lifeless, bleeding body on the road. This precious creature that just moments before had been running next to me was suddenly still and lifeless. Sitting down, hugging my legs close to me, I sobbed so deeply I felt like my heart was being torn from my chest.

When I saw any creature injured, human or animal, it caused a painful response in my own body. The feeling was even stronger when one of my brothers or my dad would cut his finger. I would bring the ointments and bandages and stand transfixed while my mother, trained in nursing, would care for the wound. I saw my brother step on a board with a rusty nail hidden that went straight through the bottom of his foot, sticking out the top. My grandfather Ira, an expert woodworker, bore the remnant of an injury years before I was born when he accidentally sawed off the first two inches of his pointer finger. Even though he would jokingly tell us grandkids that it was from picking his nose one too many times, I instinctively understood the harsh reality of the farm (and his woodworking shop). It wasn't long before I was caring for my family's injuries. My dad, my first real patient, would come home with a scraped arm or a cut finger. I would run to grab a bandage and antibiotic ointment, and he would lift me up on the counter where I would sit patiently while I put four or five bandages on his finger. I thought the more bandages I used, the more I was helping him to heal. It's ironic, but years later in medical school I learned that's sort of how mainstream medicine looks at it too: diagnose the disease and prescribe the bandage or drug of choice. Unfortunately, there is not always investigation into what caused the disease or a plan to reverse the disease process. Straight to bandage we go!

Being an HSP in my stoic "showing pain is weakness" family made me feel a bit like an outsider. I was always attuned to my family members' moods, and if they were down, I would try to be cheerful. I tried my best to try to make them laugh or smile. Thank goodness my family members still have all their appendages and that we all survived our childhood. Not all our neighbors were so lucky. More than once when I was young, a neighbor's child was killed in a farm accident, reinforcing the reality that while we had a great deal of love and support in our tight-knit community, farm life also had a harsh and unforgiving side.

"WHAT'S A VEGETARIAN?"

As I slid into my teenage years, I looked around and saw a world where everyone I knew ate meat at almost every meal. I also noticed that I didn't feel all that well after eating the steak and potatoes that made up much of the Midwestern diet. My intuition was telling me that I had the freedom to choose my own path and that my body needed something different, so I decided to become a vegetarian at the age of fourteen. In my family, not eating meat was viewed with about as much skepticism as if I'd decided not to breathe oxygen. My brothers thought I was crazy, and I'll never forget my uncle leaning across his T-bone steak to ask me, "What's a vegetarian?"

After I explained, he said, "Well, if you don't eat meat, what do you eat?"

After twenty years of practicing medicine, I now realize that I should have paid more attention to his question; there was wisdom there. My intentions were spot on, but I didn't really understand how to go about it in a healthy way. I ate a lot of processed soy products, pasta, and bread. The starches and carbohydrates were certainly not much better for my body than the meat, but I didn't know any better at the time, so as my meat intake went down, my carb intake went up.

Like any teenager, I liked the feeling of pushing back against my family norms and the idea of doing something good for my body (even though I was going about it all wrong). I had other motivations for my dietary change as well, one many young women can relate to: body image. When I looked in the mirror, I thought my tummy looked bloated and my face puffy. Even though I was a perfectly appropriately sized fourteen-year-old girl, I didn't feel well. Now I know there were a couple of culprits. Facial swelling is associated with the inflammation caused by food intolerance.[7] Unbeknownst to me at that time, my love affair with bread and pasta in place of eating meat was not a healthy relationship for my gluten-intolerant body. My tummy bloating was also likely related to my undiagnosed celiac disease, which causes fluid retention and bloating due to the small intestine being unable to absorb nutrients properly.[8] But I wasn't fat. I was inflamed. I changed my diet in part so I would look and feel differently, but I went about it in a way that caused more harm than good. What ended up almost becoming disordered eating for me in high school now makes more sense as I read *No Bad Parts* by Richard C. Schwartz, whose Internal Family Systems (IFS) theory has been transforming conventional psychology for decades. He recalls the three things he frequently saw in families of the bulimic young people that he treated when he started his career. Their families (1) believed conflict was dangerous and avoided fighting openly; (2) held disdain for vulnerability and neediness; and (3) felt the need to present a perfect image to the outside world. I could relate to these qualities in my own family, as we did our best to avoid outward conflict and present a flawless image to the world. Most of the community members in the small religious farm town where I grew up did the same.

I also used supermarket beauty products on my face and body, unaware of the damage of hormone-mimicking additives and other toxic chemicals that would further overload my little bucket. I wish I could go back and tell my younger self that she was perfect and didn't need to try to change her appearance. Unfortunately the message to young people today is even more harmful since the filtered world of social media distorts reality, creating a very unrealistic and unattainable version of beauty. Is it any wonder that both depression and plastic surgery is on the rise in women under the age of eighteen? It took me nearly a decade and a very near brush with death to begin to love myself exactly how I was.

Toxic Beauty

Many young women are unwittingly exposing themselves to massive quantities of toxic chemicals and heavy metals by using certain beauty products. Some of the worst are hormone-mimicking compounds that confuse the endocrine system during the most vulnerable time of life.

Toxins to watch out for in beauty products include:

- Parabens: Xenoestrogens are easily absorbed through the skin; adolescent girls who wear makeup daily have twenty times higher levels of parabens in their urine.[9]
- Phthalates: These are a class of chemicals associated with both cancer and reproductive toxicity—they're banned in cosmetics in Europe and Canada but are still allowed in the United States.[10]
- Fragrance: The toxicity of fragrances is only beginning to be studied, but even usually reserved researchers have labeled them as "slow poisons" and "wolves in sheep's clothing."[11] Be aware of any ingredient labeled simply as "fragrance."
- Bisphenols: BPAs are estrogen-disrupting substances found in beauty products, and absorption of them through the skin has been shown to be a significant source of toxicity.[12]
- Heavy metals: These are common in beauty products. For lead specifically, even exceptionally low levels are considered hazardous to children under six and pregnant women.[13]

Visit www.ReadUnexpected.com/Resources to find out more about how to choose healthy beauty products.

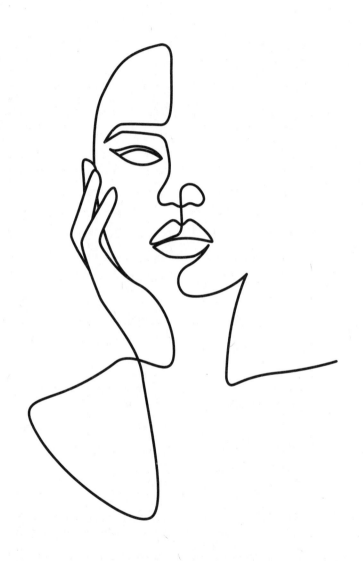

CHAPTER 3

Seek Wisdom and Embrace Uncertainty

*Let go of certainty. The opposite isn't uncertainty. It's openness,
curiosity, and a willingness to embrace paradox, rather than
choose sides. The ultimate challenge is to accept ourselves
exactly as we are, but never stop trying to learn and grow.*

—Tony Schwartz

THE NIGHTMARE

I WOKE IN A COLD SWEAT SOAKING MY NIGHTGOWN, DREAMING OF fog closing in around me, choking me with its grip like a hungry python, making me gasp for breath and clutch my chest. I looked at the time, 2 a.m., projected in red light on the bedroom ceiling. I rarely suffered from insomnia or awoke in the middle of the night. But something was wrong. There had been signs. There are always signs. Over the preceding six months when swimming laps at my medical school's indoor pool where I could usually swim 1,000 meters (about forty lengths) without a break, I had to stop every length to catch my breath. I developed a rash of cold sores around my nose that coalesced into an ugly, quarter-sized bleeding ulcer. My intuition tried to tell me that something more sinister was going on, but I pushed it aside and just chalked it up to the grueling grind of a third-year medical student's life.

Drowning in the workload, I even managed to make light of the pill-sized patch of oddly thick, firm tissue that I found on my left breast near my armpit. At twenty-four years old, I had never done routine breast exams, so I had no idea if this was new or normal breast tissue, but by this point my intuition was screaming, trying to be heard through the cacophony of med school stress. A week later I showed the lump to my husband, Aaron. I watched his eyes as his fingers probed the lump under my left arm. He tried to hide the fear that fleetingly darkened his bright blue eyes, then said, "Jilly, I think you should get this checked out right away." I shot him an exasperated look, but I knew better than to discount his intuition.

Because I was a student, after my ultrasound and mammogram I had the uncomfortable privilege of immediately reviewing the imagery with the radiologist. We sat in a dark room lit by a huge screen showing larger-than-life images of my breasts. I watched him pause, shocked by what he saw, before he explained calmly that the calcifications we were looking at would be highly suspicious of cancer in a fifty-five-year-old woman but that it was very unlikely in a twenty-four-year-old.

A few days after the biopsy and my twenty-fifth birthday, a single phone call changed my life forever. My heart pounded as I saw Dr. Smith, the oncology surgeon, appear on the caller ID. I will never forget falling into the hunter green papasan chair in our living room as I received the worst news of my life. Her voice cracked as she said, "Jill, I don't even know how to tell you this, but you have invasive ductal carcinoma; the biopsy showed that the cells that make up this cancer are very aggressive and yours has all the markers for a deadly disease."

I already knew what she wouldn't put into words, that women my age had about as much chance of winning the lottery as getting breast cancer but also that we were far more likely to die from it. I couldn't breathe. I felt the grip of the deadly fog python from my dream as the blood drained from my head and my limbs began to tingle.

"How can you be sure?" I asked, desperately hoping they had made an error in the diagnosis.

I could hear her genuine difficulty in forming the words as her voice cracked and she said, "I am so sorry, Jill."

I held it together just long enough to hang up the phone. Aaron was working an hour away. I was home alone. After a lifetime of stoically hiding my emotions, I crumbled, my mind struggling with disbelief. I observed my body as if from above as I dropped to the floor in the fetal position, sobbing from the depths of my soul, hearing tortured sounds that I had never made before. I wept until I could not produce another tear, grateful that I was alone in these first moments of processing the shock and grief of the news. Had I been with anyone else, not only would I have felt the deep shame of falling apart but I would have surely reverted to making sure they were okay (as was my habit) instead of allowing my own mind and body to begin to process the terrible news. Eventually I picked myself up and called Aaron.

He already knew. He knew from the moment he felt the lump in my left breast. In the midst of a traditional medical school curriculum, I found myself suddenly enrolled in a live-or-die private education in health care. Dr. Smith had just introduced me to my teacher, a small lump of chaotic, rapidly dividing cancer cells growing in my left breast.

"I WAS ILL, AND YOU CARED FOR ME"

During my senior year of high school my classmates voted me as "Most Health Conscious," which ended up being quite ironic, considering how my body would be ravaged by severe disease within just a few short years. I chose to major in bioengineering and minor in Spanish at the University of Illinois. By the fourth year of the bioengineering program, we were designing mechanical prosthetics and devices for medical procedures. I had no interest in mechanics—I couldn't even change the oil in my car—but I was fascinated with the human body and the science of physics and engineering. It ended up being a wonderful choice in no small part because it was one of the first years that bioengineering was offered, so very few students were enrolled in the program, and we received a lot of personalized attention. Growing up on the farm where healthy living was a core value, I knew diet and lifestyle were every bit as important as the more high-tech tools we were learning about in bioengineering classes.

> Designing a better wheelchair was a worthy goal, but I knew that helping a person stay out of the wheelchair in the first place was where true healing was found.

Our family's chiropractor, Dr. Vernon Mannon, became a most unlikely role model. He had survived polio and walked hunched over, with severe scoliosis and a post-polio limp. He had used chiropractic medicine and a deep understanding of the human body to save his own life and was the first person I heard speak knowledgeably about the value of nutrition in optimal health. Despite his hunched appearance, Dr. Mannon, with his round, jovial face and twinkling eyes, would chuckle and offer generous words of wisdom at every visit, often sitting down on the table next to me and acting as if he had all the time in the world, a pleasant contrast to the constant hustle and bustle of the Hodel farm.

On one of our visits to Dr. Mannon's office, when I was about ten years old, I noticed a tattered book on nutrition holding the place of honor at the front of his bookshelf. When he saw my gaze, he promptly took it off the shelf and suggested I take it home with me. Over the next few weeks, I savored every word of that book. It had diagrams about how food is digested, how nutrients are used by the body, and how food and lifestyle can heal almost any illness. I remember thinking, in my wonder-filled, ten-year-old mind: *Food can heal us! This is utterly amazing!*

At one point I casually asked Dr. Mannon if he thought I could be a chiropractor like him. He sat me down and very seriously told me, "Jill, you're too smart to be a chiropractor." I realize now that he meant no disrespect to chiropractors; rather, he was subtly informing me that historically his field was not respected or taken seriously by certain people, particularly medical doctors. In his many years as a chiropractor, he had suffered persecution by traditional allopathic (mainstream) physicians. This was the first glimpse I had into one of the great dichotomies of medicine: that some of the different specialties don't get along. This made no sense to me. It still doesn't. The plumber doesn't disrespect the electrician. Chiropractors, naturopaths, acupuncturists, psychologists, medical doctors, dentists, and each of us in health care professions—we're all in the job of healing people, and we each have different perspectives and skills to aid in the process, so why the conflict?

Today I work closely with, and learn from, incredible practitioners from many other healing professions. What I took from the conversation that day was that perhaps by choosing to pursue a conventional medical degree, I could make a significant change in the system from the inside out. While I certainly didn't decide to become a doctor that day, it was the conversations with him that planted the seed.

At my medical school admission interviews, I was surprised to learn that my rural upbringing was not a detriment; in fact, the administrators were intrigued by having a down-home farm girl from Illinois attending their highly respected programs. Although I had volunteered hundreds of hours at local hospitals and clinics, I didn't really expect to get accepted into medical school. I realize now this was one indication of my deep lack of self-worth that would haunt me for decades before life's challenges would teach me how to love myself. My lack of confidence was absurd. My grades had brought me the high school honor of valedictorian, my volunteer work in medical missions to Honduras gave me valuable experience, and my undergraduate coursework in bioengineering and Spanish made me well prepared for the rigors of medical school. Even so, my hands shook as I began to open the acceptance letters. Could I really become a doctor? I was the first person in my extensive line of ancestors to even consider this a possibility.

Stritch School of Medicine at Loyola University was a brand-new edifice in the Chicago suburbs with stunning architecture of modern urban glass and steel that took my breath away. Walking into those hallowed halls was the first time I believed my dream might be possible. Like many of the miracles I had witnessed in my life, I beheld this idea with equal parts wide-eyed wonder and deepest gratitude.

Standing in the glimmering atrium, I looked up at the wall to see a phrase prominently inscribed: "I was ill, and you cared for me." Growing up in a devout Christian family, I'd heard this before. I had no idea when I first entered the hallowed halls of Loyola that this would turn out to be not just an inspiration for me to use my deep empathy to care for the sick but also a foreshadowing of the compassionate care I would receive when I was diagnosed with cancer as a student there. As I read the words on the wall, my intuition told me I had found my true calling. My decision to attend Loyola was made that day.

> I knew I could make a bigger difference if I infiltrated the ranks of mainstream medicine and became a force of change for a new way: personalized, precision medicine that combined the best of both worlds.

At Loyola, I would gain the best education in medicine and be given excellent tools for dealing with acute illness and trauma. There is no better place to go after a heart attack or an auto accident than a Level 1 trauma center. However, I also knew that our country is facing an epidemic of diseases brought on by lifestyle and the environment—poor diet and nutrition, high stress, and toxic air and water—and that no pharmaceutical pill will solve that problem. I decided I could be most effective as a healer if I did my training at Loyola and then educated myself in other therapies, nutritional and lifestyle interventions, herbal medicines, and mind-body modalities to increase the tools available to reverse complex chronic illness with a personalized approach.

IN GOOD COMPANY

Oddly, I wasn't ever attached to becoming a medical doctor. I wanted to help people heal, and the "how" mattered little. There are many paths to this end, and becoming a conventional doctor was only one of them. I also knew that in allopathic medical school I would be trained in many therapeutics that, while designed to make a patient feel better, would not necessarily help the patient reverse disease processes, and at times they had unintentional side effects. A big part of my interest in a more holistic approach was driven by my belief in the interconnectedness of all things. Traditional allopathic medicine tends to discount everything outside of the pharmaceutical-focused, silver bullet approach to treating illness. But I believed in a realm where miracles were possible, where things could happen that defy scientific explanation. From the stories my father read to us in the old red living room, my childhood was steeped in miracles of those who believed in the impossible and saw outcomes that defied logic.

You may wonder how I developed such a passion for science while staying unwaveringly committed to my faith in the Divine. The truth is, I don't have a passion only for science. I have a passion for gaining wisdom through experience and understanding the "why" behind disease. I view science and faith as totally compatible parts of life.

> To me, science is the process of testing theory in order to understand the inner workings of our world and the human body. Faith is simply a peaceful relationship with the inevitable uncertainty that arises when we don't have all the answers.

I didn't know it at the time, but it turns out my perspective isn't so different from some of the early visionaries who sought knowledge about how the universe and the human body function. Robert Boyle, the man considered to be one of the founders of modern chemistry, said, "A deeper understanding of science was a higher glorification of God." James Clerk Maxwell memorized the Bible by the time he was fourteen and then went on to develop equations used to unify the forces of electricity of magnetism and to understand light as an electromagnetic wave. Even Isaac Newton himself, one of the most famous scientists of all time, spent more time on Bible study than on math and physics. He wrote:

> This most beautiful system of the sun, planets and comets could only proceed from the counsel and dominion of an intelligent and powerful Being. And if the fixed stars are the centers of other like systems, these, being formed by the likewise counsel, must be all subject to the dominion of One; especially since the light of the fixed stars is of the same nature with the light of the sun.

Gregor Mendel, the first to conduct experiments that demonstrated genetic inheritance, was abbot of a monastery in Austria.[14] More recently, Charles Townes, the inventor of the laser, winner of the 1964 Nobel Prize in physics, and professor at Berkeley until his death in 2015 wrote:

> The goal of science is to discover the order in the universe and to understand through the things we sense around us, and even man himself. This order we express as scientific principles or laws, striving to state them in the simplest and yet most inclusive ways. The goal of religion may be stated, I believe, as an understanding (and hence acceptance) of the purpose and meaning of our universe and how we fit into it. Most religions see a unifying and inclusive origin of meaning, and this supreme purposeful force we call God. Understanding the order in the universe and understanding the purpose in the universe are not identical, but they are not very far apart.[15]

More recently, Dr. Cleve Tinsley IV, humanities professor and executive director for the Center for African American History and Culture (CAAHC) at Virginia Union University, concluded in his PhD dissertation that:

> There is collaboration between science and [faith]. They really can work together, especially as it relates to medicine. This was true among both high and low social-economic status . . . there is a reality that progress in science has helped persons of faith with different issues of health.[16]

So, when I walked through the doors of Loyola University with a thirst for greater scientific knowledge and unshakable faith, I was in good company.

THE EMPATHY DESTROYER

My medical education was a stark juxtaposition between the beautiful and the inhumane. Patient interactions provided sublime honesty, miraculous healing, and countless moments demonstrating the beauty of the human soul. On the other side of the coin was a rigid culture of misogyny, work overload, and a brutal caste system. Thirty-six-hour shifts were standard fare in those days, and it was common to have just four days off per month. At the top of the residency totem pole were the attending physicians, with the senior residents just below, the interns or first-year residents below them, and finally the lowly medical students. Third-year students were the lowest of all. I was at the very bottom.

We took turns collapsing on a cot in a call room (more like a closet) when sleep overcame us. We had little time to prepare food, so my diet suffered. I'm not naturally an anxious person, but in medical school that meant they just pushed me harder, and I rarely complained, still an expert at suppressing emotion. Lewd comments and bum grabs were not uncommon. Everyone dumped "scut work," the most demeaning tasks, on those below them in rank. The term *scut* stood for "Some Clinically Useful Task," but it really meant all the unpleasant work like tracking down lab values, making sure the patient's urine was properly collected, cleaning up bodily fluids, taking blood draws, taking samples to the lab, staying up all night and retracting a wound during emergency surgery, and anything that no one else wanted to do. Retracting might seem easy, but after holding the retractor instruments under tension for six hours straight, without a chance to straighten my cramping arms or even go to the bathroom, it was physically and mentally exhausting. Even taking physical and emotional well-being out of the picture, this culture was in no way designed to create empathetic patient-centered physicians.

When I looked at the first-year medical students, I saw a group of people with hearts full of compassion and empathy. Four years later, when they walked out with their MD certifications in hand, most of them were hardened by a system that intentionally brutalizes medical students to the point that they completely shut down their own emotions.

We were taught, both explicitly and implicitly, to not connect deeply with patients; God forbid we should ever cry or show emotion in front of a patient. The reason was well-intended, like my parents' rule against naming stray dogs and cats. It hurt me to see someone in pain, so I suppose medical school was designed to remove compassion from our hearts so we could function around so much suffering.

> The problem with this approach, no matter how well-intended, is that love and connection are the antidote to pain and suffering. This is the greatest medicine of all.

We now understand how profoundly emotions affect the brain and body and that love isn't just some fluffy feel-good idea. Love and gratitude trigger the production of powerful healing chemicals, like endorphins, in our brains, and showing love triggers those around us to produce the same chemicals. These chemicals (one of which is oxytocin, sometimes called the love hormone) ease pain, boost immune function, reduce inflammation and cardiovascular disease risk,[17] increase feelings of hope and well-being, and facilitate cellular health and healing in measurable, tangible ways.[18]

Daily we saw people dying—and worse. Loyola was home to the largest burn unit in Illinois, so all the hospitals in the area sent their burn patients to us. We saw people with electrical burns and children with 80 percent of their skin gone; their eyes were so burned out you could barely tell they had a face anymore. I spent four weeks on that burn unit, and every night I'd go home exhausted and shell-shocked—you have not seen suffering until you've seen someone who has lost over 60 percent of their skin and is on a narcotic drip just to deal with the excruciating pain of drawing a breath. I would sometimes hold it together while talking to a patient and their loved ones, holding back nausea from the smell of burnt and decaying flesh, and then go to my call room to vomit. My deeply empathetic soul could not help physically feeling their pain.

This dichotomy of feeling sublime hope for difficult cases within an empathy-destroying health-care system planted the seed that would grow into my core approach to practicing medicine: love heals.

Years later, Dr. Nicole Huffman, a close friend and colleague, explained the healing potential of my love-based approach: "There are a lot of patients who are really rigid in what they believe. The same can be true for the doctor. It's important to drop the rigidity as both patient and doctor. I have seen Dr. Jill's loving approach transform patients' lives."

Simple Tips to Reduce Toxic Stress

- **Turn it down.** Limit social media and news consumption. To kick the addiction, start with turning off all media for a few days.
- **Stay present.** Do you struggle with worries about the future? Write down all your thoughts and concerns. Then put it aside, choose to let it go, and focus on the present. The present moment is all we can control.
- **Set boundaries.** Are you saying yes to that new project at work because you really want to or just because you feel that you should? One of my favorite rules is for every yes, I have to have at least five no's. This allows me to think twice before overcommitting.
- **Move your body.** We like to call it exercise, but really, it's simpler than that. Dance. Go for a walk. Make love. Hike in nature. Healthy movement doesn't have to be a fitness program. I lost stubborn body fat when I stopped strenuous exercise. This lowered cortisol, a hormone that responds to stress (and vigorous exercise!) and reduced the signal to store fat.
- **Choose to surrender.** We don't have any control over what others say or how they act, but we do have control over our own thoughts and actions.
- **Practice gratitude.** Make a list of three things that you are grateful for every night before going to bed. Meditating on these thoughts right before sleep is a powerful way to train your subconscious to look for the positive in every situation.
- **Seek sunshine.** This is a fantastic way to improve your mood and immune system with naturally occurring vitamin D.

Throughout medical school, I tried hard to keep empathy in check, but I held on to it despite all the external pressure to become hardened. I decided early on I would rather share in the suffering of my patients than be objective and remain calloused to their pain. Although it would have been easier to shut down and become numb, that empathy kept me grounded and deeply connected, teaching me some of the greatest lessons of my life as I walked with my patients in their journey to healing.

The study of empathy shows that we are endowed with "mirror neurons" that allow our brains to observe and imitate others' emotions. This is one of the paths to understanding and even diagnosing complex medical conditions. And if wisdom is gained from experience and true understanding, I don't think we can gain it without empathy. Empathy is the secret sauce for connecting with my patients on a deep level, allowing my intuition to guide me to solutions to some of the most complex medical problems.

MY LITTLE BUCKET OVERFLOWS

After working eighteen- to thirty-six-hour days, I would go home to my husband and stepchildren for a weekend of mothering and studying. Looking back, I realize I had little ability to create boundaries in my life. When I got married at twenty-one years old, I knew I was dedicating my life not only to Aaron but also to his three children. Although it was wonderful to have an instant family, I didn't know how to create healthy boundaries. I never took a day off for my own physical or mental health. I never asked someone to help make dinner because I needed a break. I didn't want to appear "weak" by asking for help. Because I never created limits for myself, I was adding a thick, toxic layer of stress and overwhelm to an already taxed sensitive system. By this time my habit of suppressing difficult emotions, like anger, fear, or sadness, was so deeply ingrained I had no idea the degree of physical and emotional stress I was actually dealing with. While I was becoming an expert in medicine, I was also becoming an expert in disassociation from my true self, especially my own needs and emotions. And I eventually learned how much this pattern contributed to the shocking diagnosis of cancer at twenty-five years old.

Many weekends I took precious days away from studying to take my three stepkids to downtown Chicago. They had never experienced urban culture mainstays like upscale restaurants or science museums, and I wanted to offer them the joy of discovery and new cultural experiences. Years later, my stepdaughter Heather told me, "You were the first woman who came into my life who was getting a college education and wasn't ashamed of being intelligent. It was the first time I had a real role model."

Unfortunately, I was also a role model for taking on way too much to be healthy or balanced. Most days, I was too preoccupied or exhausted to be present with my family. As much time as I spent with them, I was often battling other pressures like a deadline or exam or other duties in the back of my mind. Our apartment in Chicago was tiny, and when my stepson, Greg, who had Down Syndrome, would take over the loveseat and one of my stepdaughters would claim the other chair, the other stepdaughter wouldn't even have a place to sit. Aaron was away at work, and I'd be ensconced at my desk memorizing some medical minutiae that left me swinging on a pendulum between mind-numbing boredom and an urgency that the material I was studying might just save someone's life. The girls would fiddle with the stereo until I would tire of the noise interrupting my overloaded nervous system and send them down the street with a handful of spare change to get a treat from the corner store.

I thought I had to be perfect: a perfect student, a perfect stepmother, a perfect wife, a perfect daughter. Because I worked so hard at convincing everyone around me that things were perfect, my circle of loved ones never realized I needed anything. How could they? I never asked for anything, never vented my frustrations, or complained. Instead, I just smiled and did whatever anyone asked, stuffing my feelings and my needs deeper inside me with every passing day. But while I maintained my facade of perfection, those imprisoned parts of me weren't sitting idle.

Studies on melanoma patients were the first to explore the possibility of a "Type C" personality, those people with repressed coping reactions and an increased risk of developing cancer. Everyone knows about the infamous Type A individuals, those aggressive control freaks who are more prone to heart disease. The rest of us were grouped into the Type B personality category, those more balanced folks who can feel and express emotion more appropriately. But the strong associations between cancer risk and psychosocial elements gave rise to the Type C category. This person was described in an article in the *Journal of Psychosomatic Research* as "extremely cooperative, patient, passive, lacking assertiveness and accepting." Both Type B and Type C have an easygoing demeanor, but Type B is able to express anger, fear, sadness, and other emotions, while the Type C individual "repressed 'negative' emotions, particularly anger, while struggling to maintain a strong and happy facade."[19]

Meet Jill Carnahan: Type C poster girl.

Dr. Gabor Maté is one of the world's experts on the interface between stress and disease and wrote an excellent summary of my susceptibility in his book *When the Body Says No*:

> While we cannot say that any personality type causes cancer, certain personality features definitely increase the risk because they are more likely to generate physiological stress. . . . It is stress—not personality per se—that undermines a body's

physiological balance and immune defenses, predisposing to disease or reducing the resistance to it.[20]

And then there were the toxic chemicals. When I was in my early forties and saw in the headlines that glyphosate, the most popular herbicide on earth, had been contributing to cancer for decades, I decided to explore a bit deeper into the toxic layer cake that was my life twenty years earlier. I asked my dad if he remembered what chemicals he used on the farm when I was young. Incredibly, he still had his meticulously kept handwritten journal of chemicals he'd ordered for the farm. It blew my mind. My dad's chemical purchasing records from 1975 and 1976 read like a laboratory report on human toxicity. They included:

- Lasso, a Monsanto pesticide based on alachlor, a chemical categorized as a probable human carcinogen that eventually resulted in the company being sued successfully by a French farmer for chemical poisoning.
- Sutan, a butyrate-based herbicide associated with skin and respiratory irritation.
- Sencor, a herbicide based on metribuzin, a chemical that affects the thyroid gland and liver (both critical organs for the body's detoxification system).
- Aatrex, a weed killer based on the reproductive toxicant atrazine (my mom was exposed to this chemical while pregnant with me).
- And the one that really leaves me stunned: Furadan, a pesticide based on carbofuran, a reproductive toxicant and one of the most toxic pesticides ever made. The chemical is so nasty (just breathing the chemical can be fatal) that in 2009 the EPA banned the use on both domestic and imported products following a Risks and Benefits Committee report that concluded the chemical was "unduly hazardous."[21]

If you look at a map of the United States, color-coded based on application of atrazine-based farm products (like Aatrex on the list above), my home state of Illinois is dead center in the highest concentration.[22] In October 2003, two significant and opposite chemical exposure policies were announced: the EU banned the use of atrazine because of "unpreventable" groundwater contamination, and the US EPA explicitly approved of its continued use. The Centers for Disease Control information on the chemical indicates it is a proven reproductive toxicant, and some studies have shown an increase in mammary tumors in a particular strain of rats.[23]

> If someone asked me the bizarre question, "If I want to get cancer, what should I do?" I would answer by telling them to do exactly what I did.

I was born with an acute sensitivity to my environment, which I've known since I was a little girl. I always felt my detox system wasn't as robust as other people's. More recently, genetic testing confirmed my suspicion. I have multiple genetic markers associated with poor detoxification ability.

Then I went from conception through puberty on a farm soaked in atrazine (and other toxic chemicals, some of which are now banned) and developed the most aggressive form of breast cancer a person can get by the time I was twenty-five years old. When scientists classify a chemical as a carcinogen, it is typically based on animal studies showing an increased risk of cancer. But just because something isn't a known carcinogen doesn't mean it doesn't contribute to cancer development. Chemicals can also damage a person's detoxification system, which increases their susceptibility to damage from other toxicant exposure. And many chemicals act synergistically, meaning that in combination the exposures become much worse than either toxin alone. Even worse, many chemicals and drugs have their effect directly on the microbiome, dramatically altering gut health and detoxification ability.

My diet didn't help either. Since committing to a vegetarian diet when I was fourteen, I had been eating carbohydrates and processed soy every day. I didn't fully understand it at the time, but carbohydrates, especially simple carbohydrates like potatoes and white flour, convert more quickly to sugar once inside the body and create an inflammatory cellular response. My mother still loves to tell the story of asking me what my three favorite things were when I was four years old. I replied without hesitation, "God, Aunt Mary, and potatoes!" (I had a very fond relationship with my mother's younger sister, Aunt Mary, who lovingly doted on me before she had three children of her own.) While not directly responsible for my cancer, being a "carbotarian" with a soft spot for red licorice and jellybeans certainly didn't help my system resist the tumor development. There are many studies showing how sugar negatively impacts our immune system. Years later, after also being diagnosed with celiac disease, I realized that the gluten (wheat, rye, and barley) in my diet also had a major effect on weakening my immune system and creating toxic inflammation. The resulting malabsorption also left me critically depleted of vitamin B12, an essential nutrient that I later found I was sorely lacking.

The final drop in the bucket is explained through the new science of psychoneuroimmunology, the study of the mind's influence on health and disease. It's an old concept, but research into how psychological processes influence the immune system is mind-blowing. Toxins of the mind, like suppressed anger, toxic stress, and a "powerful sense of duty," are proving to significantly contribute to disease development. It's taken longer to make the connection because we can't just inject lab rats with a dose of repressed emotion the way we can with heavy metals or other chemicals, but careful research is showing that these factors are every bit as damaging as the more tangible toxins—and when it comes to breast cancer specifically, the toxins of the mind might even be more dangerous. Emotional suppression, according to a British study showing that abnormal release of emotions (like extreme suppression of anger), is the most common characteristic of breast cancer patients.[24]

SEEKING SCIENCE AND STAYING CURIOUS

I felt as if I lived an emotional lifetime between the moment Dr. Smith delivered the fateful news of my aggressive cancer and when my husband got home from work that day. When he walked in the door, we grabbed each other and sank onto the floor, cross-legged, face-to-face, holding each other and sobbing until our shirts were soaked with tears. After a few hours of stunned paralysis, the strong hand of faith pulled me out of the stew of uncomfortable emotions. I had to believe there was hope. I did the only thing my background taught me to do in the face of difficulty. I sought answers through science. Using my access to one of the best medical libraries in Chicago, I dove into the research to find a way to overcome this new challenge. The first step didn't have many options. Surgeons had to cut the tumor from my breast as soon as possible.

I had trained myself so well to never show negative emotion that, on the day when I was taken into surgery, I lay there on the gurney, joking that I would come back out of surgery lopsided. I brushed off my family's concerns, telling them it was not a big deal and that I was going to be just fine. Right before I was wheeled into the operating room, I smiled as they squeezed my hands and told them not to worry. Decades later, they all echoed the same thought: "We should have been comforting you, but you were supporting and encouraging us!"

Once the double doors closed behind me, I wept. I don't recall ever feeling so alone. It would be decades before I learned how to express my emotions to my family and friends, but I had taken the first swing at cracking my emotional shell—cancer was teaching me to express my feelings to myself, even if only when I was alone.

Once the surgery was over, the hard part began. *Radiation* and *chemotherapy* are words that are thrown around easily in the cancer discussion, but the reality is a toxic cocktail with one effect: cellular destruction. Radiation knocks out the DNA of the cell so it can't reproduce, and chemotherapy poisons the cell from the outside. Rapidly dividing healthy cells are destroyed along with the cancer. I was given a classical but highly toxic three-drug cocktail—5-FU, cyclophosphamide, and doxorubicin—that had the potential to cause heart failure, hair loss, and complete immune collapse.

I learned about a clinical trial that was applying targeted radiation to the tumor site rather than the entire chest. My concern about the standard external beam radiation was that my heart would get collateral damage from the radiation as they pointed the beams at my left breast. The good news was that the physician conducting the trial, Dr. Kuske, was located only a couple of hours away in Wisconsin. The unwelcome news was that the study group was fifty-five- to sixty-five-year-old women—twice my age and with much less aggressive forms of breast cancer. We made an appointment with Dr. Kuske anyway and spent two hours talking to him about my situation. Partway through the conversation, Aaron got down on his knees in a torrent of tears and begged, "Dr. Kuske, will you please help us, just as human beings and not subjects of your study! If you think you can help Jill, we are begging you to try!"

Dr. Kuske not only agreed to help me but also went far outside of his responsibilities as a doctor, meeting us on the weekend without staff in his clinic. After another surgeon re-excised the surrounding tissue for clean margins, he personally managed the entire radiation process for me. They surgically inserted more than twenty tubes through my left breast and then passed potent radioactive pellets through the tubes twice daily for five days. This wasn't some orthoscopic, low-impact procedure; it was a full-on skewering of my breast like some medieval torture. The idea was ingenious, though: to use physics to calculate the exact area around the tumor that needed radiation and isolate the radiation damage to surrounding breast tissues, preserving my nearby heart and lungs. In a moment of silliness, Aaron and I dubbed this experimental treatment the Shish Kaboob.

Today, a similar method, called brachytherapy, is standard practice after breast lumpectomy surgery, and I'm proud to be one of the first young women whose life was saved by it. For the past twenty years, I've been saying a blessing of gratitude every year for this forward-thinking physician, Dr. Kuske, on his birthday, which happens to fall on St. Patrick's Day. He is one of my heroes, a man who helped save my life and showed me clearly what it means to be a compassionate healer and someone willing to go outside the lines to save my life.

Once surgery was finished, it was time for toxic chemicals to target all rapidly dividing cells in my body. Chemotherapy is a nondiscriminatory treatment, and although it destroys the rapidly dividing cancer cells, it also does collateral damage to many other tissues, like the ovaries, the intestinal lining, and the hair follicles. My oncologist insisted on three-drug aggressive chemotherapy at doses that would take me right up to the limit for heart failure. I asked for it to be split into two doses over a two-day period to allow my body to better tolerate the chemical toxicity. The chemotherapeutic drugs were injected directly into my bloodstream, and the concoction was so toxic that it would have destroyed my peripheral veins, so they cut a two-inch hole in my chest and put in a central catheter to administer the drugs where the high-volume blood flow would better handle the damage. I still bear a daily reminder, like a badge of honor, a thick two-inch scar from the central line just under my left clavicle.

It has been especially important in my journey not only to discover new and innovative ways to heal from my own illnesses but to guide patients in their own healing. We can see examples of fostering life-long curiosity from intellectual greats like Thomas Edison, Albert Einstein, Leonardo da Vinci, and Richard Feynman. Albert Einstein was famously quoted as saying, "The important thing is not to stop questioning . . . never lose a holy curiosity."

> Remaining curious is one of the most important qualities of intellectual genius.

Why, you ask? In my experience, fostering childlike wonder and curiosity helps us make new discoveries in several important ways.

1. It encourages your mind to be active instead of passive. Curious people are always asking questions like "What if?" and "What else is possible?" The exercise of asking questions creates new neural pathways and enhances learning and creativity

2. It opens your mind to see innovative ideas. When you buy a new red car and suddenly start seeing red cars everywhere you go, this is called the Baader-Meinhof phenomenon, or frequency bias, when your awareness of a certain thing increases. The act of being curious opens your mind to see opportunities and ideas in everyday life that may bring awareness to solutions that were previously unseen.

3. It opens your subconscious to see new patterns and make new, innovative connections. Curiosity creates the expectation of new and unexpected ways of thinking about a problem, and creative solutions appear more easily. Your mind will automatically look for ways to connect and make meaning from unrelated concepts and will often stumble on brilliantly unique solutions to the problem at hand.

4. It adds joy and excitement in your life. Curious people by nature want to observe, try, and do new things. By engaging in novelty, the life of the curious is far from boring.

TRUSTING FAITH

Thanks to Aaron's ability to find humor in every situation, we quickly graduated from anguish to silliness whenever possible. Always a comic, whenever he saw frustration or hopelessness welling up in my eyes, he would crack a joke and usually manage to turn my tears to gut-wrenching laughter. He even managed to get the people around us caught up in the fun. When we walked into the office for my radiation treatment, Aaron would say, "We're here for my wife's shish kaboob treatment." The usually reserved nursing staff would erupt in giggles.

Rather than wait for my hair to fall out, I asked Aaron to shave my head one late summer day on the balcony of our Chicago suburb apartment. After consulting the thesaurus, I deliberately referred to myself as *glabrous*, which sounded far more glamorous than bald. We bought a pile of wigs in brunette, redhead, blond, and even pink. We had a running joke that when Aaron was on his way home from work, I would ask him which "girl" he wanted that night, the redhead, the brunette, or the blond. One evening during chemo, Aaron invited our medical school friends over for game night, and we ended the evening with everyone trying on my various wigs and laughing hysterically. Even the guys joined in, dying with laughter at their similarities to Kid Rock. When I shaved my own head, Aaron asked me to shave his head too. While we had great fun with the wigs, I only have two or three photos of me bald without a wig on. I was so self-conscious of my appearance, and although the cancer primarily affected my breasts, the far greater trauma for me was losing my hair, an undeniable outward sign that I was battling this inward demon of cancer.

Lessons from Square Watermelons

Grocery stores in Japan had a problem. Smaller than their United States counterparts, they had no room to waste. Watermelons are large and round and were wasting precious space. Instead of thinking there was nothing that could be done, Japanese farmers took a different approach. They began growing square watermelons! It turns out all you need to do is to place them in a square box and the watermelon will take on the shape of the container.

The Importance of Being Curious

- Keep an open mind. When faced with a problem, be creative in looking for a solution.
- Let go of assumptions. Just because you have done something a certain way all your life doesn't mean it can't be done better or differently.
- Ask questions relentlessly. What, why, when, where, and how are the best friends of curious people.
- Find a better solution. Seek better, more convenient ways to do something. It's impossible to find a better way if you never ask the right questions.
- Nothing is impossible. If you begin with the assumption that it can't be done, it can't. One of my favorite phrases is, "What else is possible?!" This opens the door for your subconscious to start dreaming up new and innovative solutions, sometimes even while you sleep.
- Embrace life-long learning. One of the secrets of curious people is they are lifelong learners, and most are avid readers.

Sometimes I almost forgot. But all it took was walking by a mirror and the grim reminder of my mortality and bald head brought me right back to the present.

I knew my chances of survival were grim at twenty-five, but one day while driving to my first chemotherapy appointment, my attitude changed. I heard a preacher on the radio quote John 11:4 (ESV): "This illness does not lead to death. It is for the glory of God, so that the Son of God may be glorified through it." It hit me like a lightning bolt, and I sucked in a quick breath. I turned to Aaron, who was driving, and said, "I'm going to survive this! There is an important lesson for me in this." This may have been one of the first times I heard my intuition loud and clear . . . and I clung tenaciously to this crumb of hope.

I had no idea how true that statement would become and how my choice to believe it would guide my life, but just for the moment, I felt more confident. The belief that I would survive ignited a fire within me. I told my fear to be quiet and chose instead to listen to the small whisper of hope.

This revelation further fueled my quest to understand and direct my own treatment. My oncologist didn't appreciate my curiosity, and when I asked questions about using supplements to help minimize the damage from chemotherapy, he flat out prohibited me from using any nutritional supplements. I was stunned. But I had the advantage—it was my body, my life, and my choice.

I chose to do what I knew was right for me. I realize there is great controversy around taking antioxidant supplements during chemotherapy, and I would never advise my patients to go against their doctor's recommendations, but I do believe it's important to trust your own intuition. Often in medicine we are prescribing proto-colized treatment plans for the average patient, but who is average, really? My experience in navigating my own cancer treatment set me up perfectly for a career in functional medicine precisely because there are no rigid protocols, no one-size-fits-all therapies.

> In functional medicine we use personalized and precision medicine. Every patient is treated as an individual and every therapy is personalized based on the patient's biology, physiology, genetics, and metabolism.

At first, I was convinced that I could stay in medical school and take care of my stepchildren while going through cancer treatment. Soon enough, reality hit. I was curled up in my bed, so sick that I couldn't eat, drink, or even move—let alone log a thirty-six-hour shift of scut work. My mouth and esophagus broke out in a rash of ulcers so extensive that even sipping water was painful. I reluctantly took a medical leave of absence for the duration of my treatment. This delayed my graduation by a year, but it turbocharged my education through the experience. Any time I wasn't at the hospital for treatment or sick in my bed, I read voraciously, seeking any new articles and information that might help me survive. While I certainly learned things that helped me steer my treatment, I spent a lot of time baffled by all the conflicting and inconclusive information I found. This process instilled in me a profound sympathy for the frustration felt by every patient I've seen in the years since. If looking at options for treatment was utterly confusing and overwhelming to me, a student in one of the best medical schools in the country, the feeling could only be magnified for the average patient.

Cancer therapy is not like healing a broken bone where the interventions make you feel better. Instead, the radiation and chemotherapy are so destructive that the patient suffers residual side effects from the treatment itself, sometimes for years after the cancer is gone. I lost ten pounds during treatment and Aaron gained twenty. Of the eight women who were in my support group in Chicago for women under forty with breast cancer, I was the only one who survived. Although I believed I would survive, I also knew I could just as easily have been one of the casualties. Aaron and I attended the wedding of one of the young women. It was the most beautiful and tragic love story I have ever seen—her father lifting her from her wheelchair while she said her vows to her groom and him saying "I do" with the full knowledge that his bride wouldn't live to see their first anniversary. I cried when I saw her obituary in the newspaper only nine months later.

DEVELOPING WISDOM

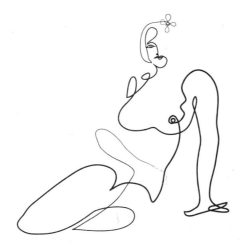

One year later I was pronounced free of breast cancer but was also weakened from the damage of chemotherapy and radiation. I was totally glabrous and weighed the same as I had at thirteen years old. I had dark circles under my eyes and the hollow but victorious look of someone who had faced death and won. I recalled the words of Edith Eger, a survivor of Auschwitz concentration camp: "Just remember no one can take away what you put in your mind." Cancer and its treatment had ravaged my body but turbocharged my passion for transforming medicine. I set about restoring my health and learning how to rebuild a body damaged by toxic chemicals designed to kill living cells. In the process, I discovered something that directed all my future.

> I wanted to become the doctor who took on the most challenging cases without fear, who would find solutions where others said there were none, who would give love and hope as a gift to each patient who walked in the door.

I wanted to work with the patient to find the root cause of a problem—to become a doctor who would buck the trends of our polarized society and practice absolute devotion to both innovative science and faith in unexpected miracles.

Just as the development of my cancer had many roots, the miracle of healing that I experienced was also multifaceted, combining the most powerful modern medicines available with nutrition and lifestyle practices, turbocharged by the abundant love that surrounded me. I certainly wouldn't have asked to endure this hardship, but cancer made me better in every way. It tested my ability as a student and became a powerful ally, showing me how to combine the faith of my youth with the science of my training, and seasoned it all with an experience that was much more than formative. These three elements—faith, science, and experience— combine to form something that medical school can't teach and money can't buy: wisdom.

When I returned to medical school, the saying written on the walls of Loyola that had drawn me to this place had never rung truer: "I was ill, and you cared for me." I was forever changed, and even my peers and professors sensed the transformation. I had been to the edge of the abyss and returned with profound wisdom. I thought my battles with life-threatening illness were over. Little did I know what was about to come next.

Lab Tests Everyone Should Consider by Age Thirty

- Complete metabolic profile
- Complete blood count with differential
- Advanced lipid panel with ApoB and Lp(a)
- Inflammatory markers: homocysteine, hs-CRP, oxidized LDL, PLAC, TMAO, and MPO
- Heavy metal testing: lead, mercury, cadmium, arsenic, aluminum
- Complete thyroid panel (TSH, free T4, free T3, TPO, TgAb, reverse T3)
- Complete hormone panel including four-point cortisol testing
- Autoimmune markers: ANA and extractable nuclear antigen panel
- Immunoglobulin levels (IgG, IgM, IgA, IgE)
- Fasting glucose, insulin, hemoglobin, A1C, and uric acid
- Serum vitamin D level
- Micronutrient testing: RBC and serum
- Celiac disease and gluten sensitivity markers
- Fatty acid testing including EPA, DHA, DPA, LA, and AA
- Iron studies including ferritin

believe

act

wait

CHAPTER 4

Believe. Act. Wait.

There are only two ways to live your life.
One is as though nothing is a miracle.
The other is as though everything is a miracle.
—ALBERT EINSTEIN

TWO NUNS ON A PLANE TO PEORIA

THERE ARE NO COINCIDENCES, ONLY INFINITE SYNCHRONICITIES. A few years ago, I was on a small commuter plane during a brief flight from Chicago to Peoria. We were jammed in so tightly that I had to check my computer bag. Two cherub-faced nuns in full habit regalia passed my seat giggling and sat down within arm's reach just one row behind me. I smiled warmly at them and wondered how their journey had led them to Peoria, Illinois, of all places.

I settled into my seat, happy to have a small coloring book stashed in my purse for just such occasions. I thumbed through the pages looking for a picture that spoke to me with just the right inspiration for the twenty-five-minute flight and chose an image of a delightful girl riding a bicycle whose countenance was full of joy. Next to her feet was inscribed a verse from Joshua 1:9 (ESV): "Have I not commanded you? Be strong and courageous. Do not be frightened, and do not be dismayed, for the LORD your God is with you wherever you go."

I chose a bright yellow sunshine-colored pencil to start. As I began to add color to the image, a small voice in my head, the same one that guides me when I'm still enough to listen, spoke clearly and plainly:

Believe. Trust in the process. Even in small things. Color the picture. Give it to the nuns.

This triggered an immediate argument from the logical part of me. My analytical mind judged the idea to be ridiculous. *What in the world would they think of me?* The self-conscious scientist in me dug in her heels and tried to ignore the thought. My intuition, the faith-filled, trusting, spontaneous part of me, was delighted with the idea but was soon overpowered by the louder, more rational voice. I let the argument recede, consumed in the therapeutic process of adding brilliant color to the picture. I colored the girl on the bicycle in a bright assortment of reds and greens and blues. I gave her golden hair and a bright smile so wide it lit up her entire face. By the time the pilot announced that we were about to descend, I was nearly finished. The voice inside spoke again, this time stronger:

Act. Give the picture to the nuns.

This reignited the argument in my head. *How ridiculous! What will they think of me?* Despite my self-doubt, this time I sided with my intuition. I gently tore the small 4 x 6 picture out of my coloring book and turned around and smiled at the sisters. I said, "Hi, my name is Jill, and I just colored this picture for you."

The sister closest to me reached out and took the picture, beaming with a huge, warm smile and a twinkle in her eye and said, "Oh my dear! Thank you!"

I could tell she was genuinely touched. A tear rolled down her cheek as she looked at the joyful girl on the bicycle and read the verse about God going with her wherever she traveled. She introduced herself as Sister Mary Rose and told me that she and Sister Cathy were flying to teach in the Montessori schools—and that the words inscribed couldn't have been any more fitting. "Sometimes travel really wears us out," she said. "We go and we go, and we serve the people we visit. We love teaching, but sometimes we get so tired, and I miss sleeping in my own bed."

I told her that I often felt the same way about my work as a doctor. We shared stories of travel and teaching and agreed on the difficulties of not sleeping in our own bed, eating various foods on the road that didn't agree with us, and all the many things that could disrupt a refreshing night's sleep. Once the seatbelt sign went off and we could get out of our seats, we stood up and hugged, laughing with joy and the unexpected connection. In a matter of minutes, I felt like I had known them for years. Sister Mary Rose printed my name on the back of the picture and said, "I will pray for you."

Now I was the one in tears. As I was walking through the airport, Sister Mary Rose asked me what kind of medicine I practiced. I softly said, "I am sure you haven't heard of it. I did my training in family medicine, but I now seek to find the root cause of disease in patients with complex chronic illness who have struggled to find answers in the current medical system. It's called functional medicine."

"Oh my!" she squealed. "I love functional medicine. I have been working with a practitioner near the monastery!"

Now it was my turn to smile. Even though functional medicine is changing the landscape of medicine, many people have never heard the term before. I handed her my card and said, "Well, if you ever need anything, will you please call me?"

We walked off the plane laughing like schoolchildren. I felt as if I were surrounded by angels. When my mother and father saw me walking out of the gate flanked on right and left by the beautiful, beaming pair of nuns in their striking black-and-white habits, they joined in the laughter. We hugged and went our separate ways, but I felt like it wouldn't be the last time I'd talk to the Sisters.

Wait for the miracle.

A year later, I received an email: "I don't know if you remember meeting two nuns on a plane to Peoria . . . but I am reaching out to see if you might be able to help me."

There are no coincidences. I believed the voice of intuition and acted upon it, even though my intellect told me the idea was foolish, resulting in an unexpected miracle. Let me take a minute to define the word *miracle* lest your first thought be, *Well, that's fine for you, but what about me? I don't even believe in God!* According to Webster's dictionary, a miracle is "an extraordinary event manifesting divine intervention in human affairs." But if we look at the second part of the definition, it includes "an extremely outstanding or unusual thing, event or accomplishment." Whether you want to call it a miracle, like I do, or just an outstanding, unexpected opportunity, either way it rings true!

The process of trusting my intuition and acting on it broke down barriers between Sister Mary Rose's habit and my jeans and T-shirt. What we were wearing didn't matter: we were sisters serving a higher purpose, each of us weary and in need of encouragement. Some of the most unexpected friendships that help us on our journey come from believing, acting, and expecting beautiful things to happen as a result. As I worked with Sister Mary Rose to help her solve her health problems, I was reminded of this simple but powerful formula that has allowed me to witness amazing opportunities and unexpected miracles throughout my life.

Believe in what is possible.

Take action.

Wait for the opportunity; wait for the miracle.

Like hopping across slippery rocks in an obscure fog, I learned that I must have the faith to leap to the rock right in front of me before the next one reveals itself. But faith alone doesn't cut it. It is a three-part equation: first, I must believe that the desired outcome is possible even if I can't see it clearly; second, I must act by jumping to the next rock, doing things like creating healthy, sustainable habits, leveraging what is in my control, doing the demanding work, studying the material, and preparing for the desired outcome; and finally, I patiently wait for the resources, the relationships, or the opportunities to manifest my miracle, moving past uncertainty into joyful gratitude as if it has already occurred.

FEVERS IN THE ER

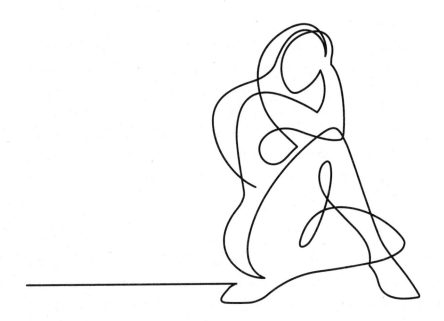

Cancer showed me the healing potential we each possess, but it was my next bout with illness that taught me to understand the healing process. I was back in medical school just a month after my cancer treatment ended. I had just begun my ER rotation, an exciting and adrenaline-filled part of medical training. Fresh off my leave from cancer, my chances of survival were looking good. I felt that empowering sense of purpose and meaning that so many survivors describe: a more profound appreciation and understanding of life.

Susan Cain deftly describes this in her book *Bittersweet*, saying it is precisely during times of impermanence, like career changes, divorce, or facing life-threatening illness or death, that we are more likely to experience meaning, communion, and transcendence. Researchers found that two items consistently appeared as major triggers to this feeling of transcendence: transitional periods of life and being close to or facing death. "In other words," says Cain, "during any period of the intense awareness of passing time—the hallmark of bittersweetness itself."[25] She goes on to say that bittersweetness is about the recognition that light and dark, birth and death, bitter and sweet, are forever paired. We really cannot experience one without the other. Although I never fully grasped the power of bittersweet prior to reading her book, I secretly smiled at the thought that one of my favorite places to write and meet friends in my hometown of Louisville, Colorado, is called Bittersweet Café.

Overcoming cancer gave me new passion for paving the way for a new model of practicing medicine. I had taken nine months off for the brutal cancer treatment, and although my will was strong, my body was still recovering from the effects of chemotherapy and radiation. But something new was wrong. I was still underweight from the cancer treatments, but I should have begun gaining weight back. Instead, I continued losing weight and was experiencing episodic abdominal pain that made me curl into a ball. At first I thought it was just residual pain from the damage of chemotherapy and radiation. Surely, the painful symptoms would pass. But then I began having cyclical fevers each afternoon. My mind was in complete denial that anything was seriously wrong, but once again my intuition already knew.

As medical students, unless we were admitted to the hospital, we were expected to report to work. I showed up for each shift, helping all manner of patients who presented to the emergency room—the whiplash injuries and trauma after car accidents; the sunken, yellowed eyes and swollen bellies from alcoholic liver failure; the acute respiratory distress from pneumonia or pulmonary edema; and sadly, on occasion, the distressing calls after domestic violence and the inevitable fabricated story. My curiosity was still unquenchable, and every patient taught me something new about the art of healing. The ER was one of the most common places for doctors to become calloused to immense suffering. It was hard not to squelch the empathy as the pain and suffering encountered there was sometimes overwhelming. In focusing my heart on helping the most critical patients, I ignored the terrible symptoms manifesting in my own body, right up until they knocked me down. Literally.

Severe abdominal pain. Fevers up to 102 degrees. "I'm just fine, thank you."

One day while examining a patient, feeling a bit lightheaded from the fever, I suddenly passed out cold. There's nothing quite like waking up on the floor of the emergency room while you're supposed to be helping the sick and injured. A couple of days later, I found myself on the other side of the stethoscope.

The doctor became the patient. Again. Sigh.

There was an abscess in my bowel that needed immediate drainage and surgery. When I awoke from emergency surgery, still groggy from the anesthesia, the attending surgeon delivered the news. I had Crohn's disease, a severe autoimmune condition in which the body attacks the gut lining, creating malabsorption, inflammation, and severe damage to the gastrointestinal tract. He explained that he had drained and packed the abscess and started me on antibiotics. He said my fevers would improve, but based on his experience, I would be learning to live with this new diagnosis.

In hindsight, I realize that the combination of experiencing cancer and Crohn's disease during medical school was the ultimate blessing as a physician in training. Like learning a new language in an online course but then moving to a foreign country to practice it, my understanding of the physical and emotional aspects of illness were enhanced immeasurably. There were deep insights and understandings that I never could have learned while sitting in the lecture hall or reading a textbook. While I could have succumbed to anger, shock, or overwhelm, I chose none of these. Instead, I believed that there was purpose and meaning in the struggle. I chose to believe there was a treasure to be found hidden within each experience of adversity that I encountered.

> This perspective pushed my fear and sadness aside with an equally powerful set of emotions: hope and curiosity, my secret to experiencing unexpected miracles.

My dear friend, brilliant physician, and best-selling author Sara Gottfried has seen the power of curiosity fuel healing in her own body as well as in the bodies of her patients, and she explains beautifully how the greatest feats of healing she's seen often happen when the patient sees a diagnosis as an opportunity and says, "Oh look, there's something happening to my body. What is it here to teach me?"

This opportunistic view describes how I've always approached suffering. The experience of Crohn's was more mysterious than the better understood cancer I had just survived, but I knew there was something within the experience that would make me a stronger woman and a more capable healer. What about you? What is your struggle? Is it possible to become curious instead of bitter and look for the wisdom held within the experience?

PERFECTLY "INCURABLE"

As I learned more about the triggers to autoimmune disease, I realized that the dysfunction is caused by three primary factors. The good news was that I had some control over at least two of them. Autoimmunity simply means that the body is mistaking its own tissues as a dangerous stranger and the immune system attacks. Really, it is a simple case of mistaken identity. There are at least eighty named autoimmune diseases, including Crohn's, but all autoimmunity has three things in common. Originally called the triad of autoimmunity by Dr. Alessio Fasano in 2012, the three factors are 1) genetics, 2) environmental and infectious triggers, and 3) intestinal permeability, or leaky gut.[26]

The second part of the triad, environmental or infectious triggers, can be a wide range of culprits, including foods such as gluten, dairy, egg, soy, corn, sugar, peanuts, and lectins. In addition, heavy metals, other toxicants, pesticides, and even naturally occurring environmental toxins like mold or infections (bacteria and viruses) can trigger an autoimmune reaction. We have seen this clearly with SARS-CoV-2 and its tendency to trigger other autoimmune diseases in certain people.[27]

The third, and the most recently discovered part of the triad of autoimmunity, is intestinal permeability, or leaky gut. This occurs when the tight junctions between the cells that line the intestines become more porous or permeable, allowing larger molecules to enter the bloodstream. The tight junctions, controlled by zonulin, which acts like a physiological traffic cop that controls traffic across the cells that line the gut. I often describe these cells like tiles on your bathroom wall. Similar to grout that has been damaged or cracked, the junctions between the cells may lose their integrity and allow for the passage of molecules that would normally not be allowed to pass through. It's like having Swiss cheese for a gut lining. Some particles, like bacteria or partially digested food proteins can then pass directly into the bloodstream. The immune system goes to work creating antibodies to anything it deems a dangerous stranger, and sometimes these antibodies react to our own tissues, creating an autoimmune condition. This is called molecular mimicry.

With this knowledge, I had the hopeful realization that if I could identify and reduce the environmental triggers, like food, bacteria, or fungi, and begin to restore the integrity of my intestinal lining, I might be able to heal from my Crohn's disease.

After I recovered from the surgery, I had an appointment with a new gastroenterologist to discuss a treatment plan and answer any questions I might have regarding my new diagnosis. After listening politely to him explain my diagnosis, I had one final question: "Could diet have any influence on my condition?" My memory of his reply is as clear as if it happened yesterday:

"Jill, diet has nothing to do with it."

I intuitively knew he was wrong then, but it took me years to learn just how wrong. And the myriad literature since my diagnosis in 2002 supports my current understanding. Seventy percent of the immune system is found in the lining of the intestines; autoimmune diseases have *everything* to do with diet. He also told me that my condition was "incurable" and that I would likely need drugs to modulate my immune system for the rest of my life and should prepare myself for multiple surgeries over time to remove damaged parts of my colon. I walked out of the gastroenterologist's office, firing the second of my doctors in less than a year, but I am grateful for the experience. He had just taught me one of the most important lessons of medicine: empower the patient. Ever since then, my primary goal as a physician has been to inspire the patient to partner with me in creating a treatment plan.

> The patient knows themselves better than anyone, and they are the sole owner of an important key to a healing reserve of immense potential: the subconscious mind.

At the moment I walked out of his office, I didn't know exactly how to heal from Crohn's disease, but intuitively I knew there had to be a way. To find the solution, I needed to dig all the way to the root of the problem. Distilling twenty years of research and the results of my own genetic testing into a couple of paragraphs, here's what I believe happened:

Testing confirmed that I was born with a genetic predisposition for Crohn's disease. I carry a mutation in a gene called NOD2. This gene provided instructions to make certain proteins, which are important for immune function. These specialized proteins play a critical role in defending the body against foreign invaders, particularly recognizing certain bacteria and stimulating the immune system to respond. The NOD2 protein turns on a protein complex called nuclear factor-kappa B (NFkB), which regulates multiple immune and inflammatory reactions in the body. I've often taught about the genetics of Crohn's disease and described it as "an abnormal response to normal microbiome bacteria," meaning that my genetic predisposition created a response to bacteria that was more aggressive than normal, leading to collateral damage of the surrounding tissue.

Each one of us has specialized proteins that live on the outer surface of every cell in our body and make up what's called the human leukocyte antigen (HLA) system. These cells are the early warning system for trouble and communicate the presence of a pathogen or other invader to the heavy artillery of the immune system, the macrophages, and T cells (made famous by COVID-19 for their ability to defend against viruses) and other defensive cells.

Imagine these cells like characters in the iconic video game Pac-Man as they cruise around in the body gobbling up all the little bits that could cause you harm. In the gut lining, these cells are constantly sampling the environment as it passes through the body: "Oh, there's a piece of corn protein, that's okay" or "Ooh, salmonella—kill it. Alert the troops and notify the immune system."

In my body, this system overreacts to less dangerous triggers, like normal bacteria in the gut, and these HLA sensors become alarmed when they detect perfectly normal bacterial parts leaking into my bloodstream from the intestine. This then triggers the immune system to create antibodies and begin to attack. The inflammatory reaction often hurts perfectly normal cells that line the gut, causing massive collateral damage and the classic lesions of Crohn's disease. This condition is aggravated when the cells that line the gut, called enterocytes, are inflamed or damaged by other factors like chemotherapy. Chemotherapy drugs are designed specifically to target rapidly dividing cells, which include cancer cells but also hair follicles and the cells that line the gut.

One of the chemotherapy drugs used on my cancer is called cyclophosphamide, and one method of action is to induce leaky gut, activating the full power of the immune system against cancer.[28] When this drug punched holes in my intestinal lining, my system was flooded with a mishmash from my intestinal tract, including partially digested nutrients, bacterial coatings from my microbiome (the infamous lipopolysaccharides [LPS]), and anything else big enough to fit through the holes. This onslaught of foreign substances in my bloodstream sent my immune system into overdrive and, in theory anyway, tricked my immune system into attacking the cancerous cells in my breast. After cancer treatment, I still had a permeable intestinal lining and an overactive immune system—the perfect scenario for Crohn's to develop in someone like me with underlying genetic susceptibility.

In one sense, my gastroenterologist was correct—food may not have been the trigger that *initiated* Crohn's disease in my body, but dietary factors may have *sustained* the immune dysfunction. Unbeknownst to me, I also had undiagnosed celiac disease, so every time I ate gluten, which is found in wheat, rye, and barley, I was telling my Pac-Men to send out the alarm and increase inflammatory cytokines (immune system messengers) that caused damage to the intestinal lining. One of the most important things I did just after my diagnosis of Crohn's diseae was to eliminate inflammatory foods, like gluten, dairy, and sugar to calm down the inflammatory immune response and silence the Pac-Men. Changing my diet was a critical first step to healing.

In my search for answers, I came across a food-based approach called the specific carbohydrate diet (SCD), made famous by Elaine Gottschall in her book *Breaking the Vicious Cycle: Intestinal Health Through Diet.* The diet was originally developed by pediatrician Sydney Haas to treat celiac disease, but Elaine came across it when Dr. Haas treated her daughter successfully for severe ulcerative colitis. The very day I read her book on the SCD, I began changing my diet to remove the carbohydrate triggers that were fueling the inflammation. In just two weeks, some of my worst symptoms subsided and I knew I was on to something important. Within that time, the cells lining my intestines had been replaced four or five times, transforming my war-torn intestinal wall with a robust and functional layer of cells. It took years of modulating my immune system, repairing my gut, and changing my microbiome to consider myself cured of Crohn's, but the improvement after just two weeks of changing my diet made me feel like I'd sipped from the fountain of youth.

Although it was controversial years ago when I was diagnosed, data now supports the positive effects of dietary changes on inflammatory bowel disease. In 2017 a review of research on the SCD diet used in treating Crohn's disease concluded the diet showed promise in treating both adults and children. And in 2020 a randomized diet-controlled trial in children with Crohn's disease showed healthy microbiome shifts and decreased disease activity among all patients in a twelve-week period.[29]

Crohn's is still considered incurable by the mainstream medical community, but I have no further signs or symptoms of the disease. Many of my patients can tell you the same thing about their own bodies after applying a functional medicine approach to inflammatory bowel disease or other autoimmune condition.

Specific Carbohydrate Diet (SCD)

How the Diet Works

The theory behind the SCD diet is that certain carbohydrates remain in the small bowel where bacteria can metabolize them, leading to overgrowth of bacteria and fungi, damaging the villous mucosal lining, and producing metabolic waste products that contribute to inflammation. By limiting the carbohydrates to only those that are easily broken down, there are minimal undigested particles to create inflammation in the small bowel.

Foods Allowed on SCD Diet

- Fresh, unprocessed meat, poultry, fish, shellfish, and eggs
- Certain legumes, including dried navy beans, lentils, split peas, raw cashews, and all-natural peanut butter and lima beans
- Dairy limited to hard cheeses such as cheddar, Colby, Swiss, and dry curd cottage cheese
- Homemade yogurt fermented at least twenty-four hours
- Most fresh, frozen, raw, or cooked vegetables and string beans
- Fresh, frozen, or dried fruits with no added sugar
- Most nuts and nut flour
- Most oils, teas, coffee, mustard, cider or white vinegar, and juices with no additives
- Honey as sweetener

Prohibited Foods on SCD Diet

- Sugar, molasses, maple syrup, sucrose, processed fructose, including HFCS and any processed sugar
- All grains, including corn, wheat, wheat germ, barley, oats, and rice. This includes bread, pasta, and baked goods with grain-based flours
- Canned vegetables with added ingredients
- Legumes not mentioned above
- Seaweed and seaweed by-products
- Starchy tubers such as potatoes, sweet potatoes, and turnips
- Canned and processed meats
- Canola oil and commercial mayonnaise
- All milk and milk products high in lactose, such as commercial yogurt, cream, sour cream, and ice cream
- Candy, chocolate, and products that contain fructooligosaccharides

For more information, see Elaine Gottschall, *Breaking the Vicious Cycle: Intestinal Health Through Diet* (Baltimore, Ontario: The Kirkton Press, 1994).

> This is one of the most significant misunderstandings in medicine: incurable doesn't mean healing is not possible. It simply means there is not a drug that reverses the condition.

Healing my gut and avoiding a life of surgery and drugs started with switching to an anti-inflammatory diet, primarily plant-based and grain-free. The Crohn's-inspired life changes improved my overall energy levels. My allergies decreased significantly. Now visiting my family's farm in Illinois rarely triggers the severe allergies I had as a child. My little detox bucket now has more margin to better handle other things, like the dust, mold, and chemical residues on the farm that used to make me sick.

The dietary solution I stumbled onto has helped countless patients since then. Toxicity isn't only found in the external environment (exotoxins); it's also created inside us (endotoxins), so healing from toxicity is about controlling the external environment, certainly, but also about rebuilding the internal environment into a more resilient, less inflamed place.

I also emerged from my experience with Crohn's disease with a deeper understanding of medicine. Using diet to begin healing from Crohn's right on the heels of recovering from cancer was powerful inspiration. I wanted to help patients experience the same thing: to develop a personalized healing plan that would help them become the most resilient version of themselves.

CONFLICT OF INTEREST

I was a walking success story of the power of combining the best of conventional medicine and alternative medicine, but I disliked that term. To me it was just good medicine, period. Because I felt strongly that we should be exposed to other healing modalities, I founded an integrative medical student group, the first of its kind at Loyola. We organized evening lectures, bringing in experts from other schools to instruct the students and faculty. I invited massage therapists and acupuncturists and naturopaths and others to speak and discouraged the use of the term *alternative* to describe these other modalities of healing. I would say, "Alternative to what? It's not an alternative! We are inferring that allopathic medicine is always superior, and it's not—it's just more commonly reimbursed by the insurance system in the United States." Twenty years (and an opioid crisis and COVID-19 pandemic) later, time has shown that allopathic treatments are certainly not always better, nor are they the only answer to our declining state of health.

In the 1990s and early 2000s we began using the term *complementary medicine*, which was better, but it still failed to capture healing as one beautiful whole. Then *integrative medicine* brought it all together conceptually. I liked that, but it still left the walls between specialties, leaving the patient to navigate a world in which they were unprepared to understand or to select what was right for them.

When I first heard Dr. Jeffrey Bland speak about functional medicine, I was spellbound. He was describing the very type of medicine I had experienced in my own healing and wanted to practice.

He explains in the opening chapter of his book *The Disease Delusion*,

> The last century was all about conquering acute infectious disease, a mission largely accomplished with antibiotics, whose efficacy was expanded into an overarching "single pill for an ill" paradigm. In the 21st century, however, chronic illnesses— heart disease, diabetes, cancer, arthritis, digestive disorders, dementia, autoimmune disease, etc.—are what deprive us of our health and kill us, slowly. Even the health of our children is rapidly deteriorating. Conditions that appeared only in adults (e.g., obesity, type 2 diabetes) are now regularly seen in children, so much so that this generation is predicted to be the first whose lifespan will be shorter than that of their parents. …What is required is a new model of care capable of personalizing treatment to the individual's unique genetics, environment, diet, and lifestyle: functional medicine.[30]

From the first moment I heard Dr. Bland describe functional medicine, I knew this was my calling.

Following medical school, I began working as a family medicine physician, prescribing antibiotics, delivering babies, and helping people with myriad common health issues, from diabetes to hypertension to arthritis and everything in between. I loved my work and enjoyed the relationships with patients. But I didn't love how limited we were in our healing toolbox. I tried to help my patients determine the root cause of their symptoms, but with fifteen-minute windows to work with, my suggestions were little more than a quick footnote to the standard quick diagnosis before sending the patient out the door with a prescription. My love of medicine was tainted by my frustration at not being able to do more with the limited time I had with patients. After a day of writing prescriptions, I'd go home and consume my own medicine in the form of healthy foods that would heal and nourish my body. My health was improving every day, but many of my patients continued to struggle with their own issues. I became disillusioned with a system that seemed to be failing my patients.

> I knew taking a root cause approach to healing chronic diseases had the potential to transform our current medical system in the very best way.

For patients with diagnoses like chronic fatigue syndrome, irritable bowel syndrome, or rheumatoid arthritis, I knew no drug could completely reverse the course of the disease. However, I also knew their symptoms and quality of life could be dramatically improved with a functional medicine approach. So I would suggest they schedule a longer follow-up appointment to discuss if we should do additional testing to identify the root cause of their issues, and I'd help them incorporate lifestyle and dietary changes and other treatments to improve their health.

I saw arthritis patients who were on powerful immune-modulating medication; six months after my consultations they happily reported, "Doctor, I don't need any of this medicine anymore." I saw a patient with ulcerative colitis whose symptoms were not well controlled. When he came to my clinic, I did extensive testing on the gut microbiome and implemented a plan to treat his inflammation. A few months later, he came back to my office and said, "Doc, my symptoms are completely gone." I checked his labs, and all of the inflammatory markers were now normal.

When incredible successes started happening over and over, I was initially shocked. Of course, I hoped for some improvement in my patients, but the numerous 180-degree turnarounds I witnessed in those first few years were beyond my wildest expectations. At first when patients would come in after a few months of treatment telling me how much better they were feeling, I recall thinking, "Really!? It worked!?

> I was amazed to see the success of this functional medicine model of science-based systems biology and personalized, precision medicine in reversing disease.

After several months of offering functional medicine consultations, I had a six-month waiting list for these extended appointments. The CEO of the hospital I worked for started paying attention. After years of subduing my more intuitive healer side to follow the well-established path of allopathic medicine, the voice of intuition told me it was time to be a force of change.

So I pitched the idea of building an Integrative Medical Center to the hospital CEO.

Wouldn't you know it? He loved the idea and agreed!

One of the most exciting moments of my life was sitting with the hospital's architects and dreaming up the design for the Methodist Center for Integrative Medicine (MCIM), the first of its kind in central Illinois. We designed the facility to reflect an atmosphere of healing and aesthetic beauty. We decorated it with fine art from local photographers and artists, created a waterfall behind the front desk, and installed crown molding and recessed lighting to create a beautiful ambience that fostered warmth and healing. It also included a retail pharmacy so patients could pick up supplements or medications at their appointment, a service almost unheard of at the time. The day I cut the ribbon at the opening ceremony as the medical director of the new facility, it felt like more than just the opening of a new building. I felt a new era of medicine was being ushered in.

And for me it was just another example of the power of Believe-Act-Wait. Unbeknownst to me, however, this process also set me on a collision course with the hospital and on track to be a changemaker and leader in functional medicine.

The greatest joy was when patients no longer needed to see me or take prescription medication. After I had been running the MCIM successfully for several years, I was sitting in a board meeting with the other hospital department heads. The chief financial officer fired up a presentation that demonstrated how many beds in the hospital each department was filling, as if we were a car dealership and each bed was a new car sold. Although it wasn't stated explicitly, it was clear that the departments that filled the most beds were applauded. My integrative medicine facility was at the bottom of the list. Clearly I was succeeding at keeping patients out of the hospital.

The medicine I was practicing was healing people at least as effectively as any other department, but that's not how it was presented. I heard the implicit message loud and clear: I wasn't fulfilling the administration's expectations. Although I didn't change anything right away, I knew my days as the director of the MCIM were numbered. The new approach just didn't fit into an old, outdated model.

MOUNTAIN LIONS IN THE PARKING LOT

When my husband was offered a job in Colorado, I put my philosophy of Believe-Act-Wait into practice once again. I believed there was a future for me in functional medicine. I acted by resigning from my job as medical director of the Integrative Medicine Center and proceeded to sell our home and everything in it, moving halfway across the country from Illinois to Colorado. Then I waited patiently for the opportunity, or miracle, but not for long.

Shortly before moving to Colorado, I met Dr. Robert Rountree, or "King Bob" as he is affectionately known. He has a private consultative practice in the foothills of Boulder, Colorado, and is considered one of the visionary leaders in the functional medicine movement. His deep understanding of root cause medicine resonated with me, and so I walked up to him after a lecture, shook his hand, and said, "Hi, Bob, my name is Jill Carnahan. I'm moving to Colorado, and I think you need a medical partner." He laughed and said, "Let's have dinner and talk about it."

Dr. Rountree generously offered to share his small clinic space with me, starting one day a week. It was a tiny office nestled so close to the wilderness of the Rocky Mountains that I saw mountain lions prowling the parking lot. I had to start from scratch building a medical practice where no one knew my name, but Dr. Rountree supported me not only by sharing his space but also by sharing his razor-sharp sense of humor, confidence-inspiring wisdom from years of practice, and deep devotion to lifelong learning. I will be forever indebted to his kindness in helping me get a fresh start in Colorado.

Over the next two years, I took a massive pay cut, drained my savings, and spent every penny of the profits from the sale of our house in Illinois to start a new practice of my own. However, the move across the country delivered unexpected rewards, including the opportunity to recalibrate my life. As Eleanor Roosevelt once said, "You gain strength, courage, and confidence by every experience in which you really stop and look fear in the face. You can say to yourself, 'I have lived through this. I can take the next thing that comes along.' You must do the thing you think you cannot do."

This huge change was quite scary for me, but I believe the adventurous flavor of fear and choosing to face it anyway can be a positive influence that drives us to do some of our greatest work and allows us to live out our dreams. The fact that it was completely up to me to provide an income with no guarantees drove me to begin sharing my story publicly, both online for the first time and in giving free lectures at local health clubs and natural grocery stores. While I had previously considered myself a private person, I now realized the power that my own story of healing from breast cancer and Crohn's disease had to encourage and inspire others. I could no longer keep it to myself.

I was also stretching the bounds of my upbringing farther than anyone in my family had ever done. Just becoming a doctor was a radical concept. When I quit my secure, well-paying job as a medical director and moved to a hippy town in the mountains, some of my family thought I was crazy. While walking along Pearl Street in Boulder, I kept running into an odd, skunky aroma and finally asked Aaron, "What's that smell?"

He replied, "That's marijuana, Jill."

Farm girl was a long way from home.

Everything You Need to Know about Intestinal Permeability

At the time of this writing, intestinal permeability, or leaky gut syndrome, is not an officially recognized medical diagnosis. The Canadian GI Society published an article in 2013 "debunking the myth of leaky gut,"[48] but as recently as August 2019 in *Gut*, Dr. Michael Camilleri stated, "There is no controversy regarding barrier dysfunction in diseases resulting in intestinal inflammation and damage such as celiac or Crohn's disease, or ulceration from nonsteroidal anti-inflammatory drugs (NSAIDs) resulting in structural abnormalities of the epithelium.[49]

In functional medicine we've seen intestinal permeability as a contributing factor in serious disease for some time. Emerging research supports what we've long suspected—that intestinal permeability is a root cause of many diseases. In 2020, a bombshell article was published in *Gastroenterology*, the journal of the American Gastroenterological Society, which showed that people diagnosed with Crohn's disease had shown evidence of intestinal permeability more than three years *before* the diagnosis. The researchers concluded, "Increased intestinal permeability is associated with later development of (Crohn's disease); these findings support a model in which altered intestinal barrier function contributes to pathogenesis."[50] In the past two years, many articles have begun to be published on the connection between severe COVID-19 and increased intestinal permeability; one from 2021 in *Frontiers in Immunology* stated, "We found that severe COVID-19 is associated with high levels of markers of tight junction permeability and translocation of bacterial and fungal products into the blood."[51]

Symptoms of Increased Intestinal Permeability
- Chronic diarrhea
- Gas and bloating
- Nutritional deficiencies: fat-soluble vitamins, iron, and B12
- Fatigue
- Headaches
- Mood changes
- Brain fog
- Skin conditions: rashes, eczema, acne
- Joint pain

Causes of Increased Intestinal Permeability
- Drugs, like chemotherapy
- Excess alcohol consumption
- Parasitic infections
- Celiac disease
- Bacterial or fungal overgrowth
- High stress
- Surgery
- Severe infection or sepsis

Tips to Heal a Leaky Gut
- Eliminate gluten, dairy, and processed sugar from your diet
- Reduce stress
- Take vitamins A and D
- Take zinc carnosine
- Take L-glutamine powder
- Use bovine immunoglobulins or colostrum
- Take a spore probiotic

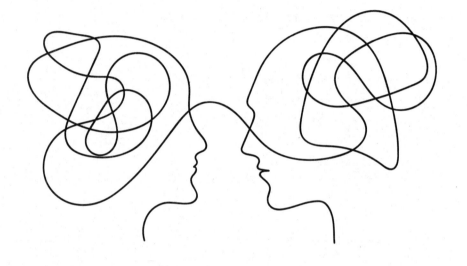

CHAPTER 5

Supercharge Healing through Flow

Motivation is what gets you into this game; learning is what helps you continue to play; creativity is how you steer; and flow is how you turbo-boost the results beyond all rational standards and reasonable expectations. That, my friends, is the real art of impossible.

—STEVEN KOTLER, AUTHOR OF *THE ART OF IMPOSSIBLE*

THE WARRIOR PRINCESS

Shivering a bit to ward off the chill from the cool air flowing down from the snowcapped peaks near my home, I pulled my hoodie a little tighter, pondering all I had just been through as I recited my new mantra: *I am Sasha, Warrior Princess, daughter of the King, worthy of great love, full of joy, conquering all fear. I will overcome all obstacles; I will outlast all adversity; things are turning in my favor.*

I had recently started taking walks along the dirt road behind my condo near a beautiful horse farm, using this as a reminder of my core values to transform my fears into the belief that greater things were to come. I was deliberately choosing this alter ego as a new identity. By calling myself Sasha, it helped me envision a stronger, more vibrant version of myself, one I always knew I could become.

I was initially shocked to realize that for many of my new neighbors in Colorado, taking considerable time away from work was normal. Coming from a farm family who routinely pulled fourteen- to sixteen-hour days at least six days per week, and after working a schedule of eighty- to one hundred-hour weeks at the medical clinic in Peoria, I initially had to stave off the guilt of not working insane hours.

For decades, Boulder, Colorado, has been high on the list of the healthiest and happiest towns in America. Recreation access certainly helps, but the biggest factor is that the community is made of tens of thousands of individuals who strive every day to make their environment as inspirational, joyful, and resilient as possible. The collective expansion of the community's embrace of health is irresistible. It's hard not to pay attention to what you eat when restaurants and stores present you with options based not just on what it will taste or look like but on how the food will treat your body. Instead of traditional fast-food chains, I was more likely to drive by an IV vitamin clinic, a local farm-to-table restaurant, or an organic green juice place on my way to work. Walk outside on a winter morning after a fresh snow, and you may find the bike paths plowed before the roads. My favorite was when I asked someone, "What do you do?" Instead of telling me how they make an income, they were more likely to respond with, "I'm a cyclist" or "I'm a rock climber" or "I love snow skiing."

This quality of my new home, where recreation was viewed with at least as much reverence as vocation, made it painfully clear to me that my own life was out of balance. The way out was understanding a problem I had always viewed as one of my greatest strengths: I didn't know how to stop working!

WILL WORK FOR LOVE

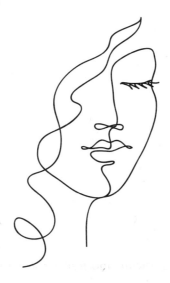

My addiction to work was deeply rooted in my Swiss-German DNA, but I never really thought of it as harmful until one day while I was attending an exclusive mastermind event. I found myself in a room full of some of the world's most successful entrepreneurs and thought to myself, *What in the world am I doing here?* Legendary CEO Joe Polish got up and started talking, straight from his heart, about his journey of overcoming addiction. He suggested we view addicts differently, with great compassion, because addiction is simply a way for us to deal with the underlying pain of unresolved trauma. When I heard the word *addiction*, I tuned it out, thinking it wasn't relevant to me. That is until he said, "Most of you in this room are addicts. You have simply chosen the socially acceptable addiction of work or performance, which reinforces the addiction because you are rewarded with recognition or financial success. It feeds your addiction to avoiding pain by seeking love through performance."

Ouch! Now he had my attention. Here I was sitting among successful health-care entrepreneurs whom I admired, and it dawned on me: many of us were being driven to succeed, to overcome, to show the world we were "good enough" or "strong enough" by the very same unresolved trauma that drove an addict to pick up the bottle or shoot up heroin. But with this addiction to achievement comes a risk just as serious as a narcotic addiction: the danger of losing oneself. I was at the threshold of doing just that. So much for thinking the discussion didn't pertain to me.

I realized that the quest to become the best in my field was holding me captive just as strongly as any addiction. Of course, it was an addiction that my family and friends had no idea I was facing, but the quest for external validation can be a heady narcotic, and it left me empty and waiting for my next fix. As I sought insight and understanding to facilitate change, I began to rebuild my environment to include stronger boundaries to protect my sensitive system, but not impenetrable walls. I needed to be able to receive love and assistance and to forge new neural pathways that lead away from the achievement-focused version of love. I was just starting to understand that I was worthy of love just for being me and not only for accolades and accomplishments. It was a humbling realization but the beginning of true freedom. That day changed my perspective.

> No longer did I think successful
> people were a superhuman species.
> Instead, I recognized they are regular
> people who have found a socially
> acceptable way to deal with the
> suffering and pain from their past.

I learned that I am no different and had been using accomplishment to feel worthy of love. I went home from that event with a newfound understanding and started looking for ways to overcome my own addiction and misaligned definition of love. But where to start?

CHASING FLOW STATES

Having spent a big part of my life as both patient and doctor, I saw clearly that our view of healing as being something that is done only when we're injured or sick is flawed. Instead, healing is a performance that our bodies do every day of our lives. We just need the tools to tap into our innate ability to heal. It was time to take a lesson from some of the most talented people on earth: athletes and creative artists. But my goal, instead of excelling at a sport or an art form, was to help myself and my patients experience daily life in the most vibrant and joyful way possible.

I wasn't so interested in the training methods of elite athletes but in the intentional manipulation of the neurochemistry of performance—specifically, the power of flow. Steven Kotler is the founder and director of the Flow Research Collective and has dedicated his life to the study of flow. In his seminal book on performance, *The Art of Impossible*, Kotler defines flow like this:

[Flow] refers to those moments of rapt attention and total absorption when you get so focused on the task at hand that everything else disappears. Action and awareness merge. Your sense of self vanishes. Time passes strangely. And performance—performance just soars.

Flow's impact on both our physical and mental abilities is considerable. On the physical side, strength, endurance, and muscle reaction times all significantly increase while our sense of pain, exertion, and exhaustion all significantly decrease.

Yet the bigger impacts are cognitive. Motivation and productivity, creativity, and innovation, learning and memory, empathy and environmental awareness, and cooperation and collaboration all skyrocket—in some studies as much as 500 percent above baseline.[31]

It was the original work of Mihaly Robert Csikszentmihalyi, who passed away as I was writing this book, that got me thinking about healing as a performance pursuit—and flow as medicine. When skiing in fresh powder and losing track of time, coloring for hours in my coloring book at the coffee shop, or dancing with unrestrained joy to the music in my headphones when I am all alone, I experience flow. But it's not just for pleasure. This same flow state also happens when I'm in my clinic. No matter what else is happening in my life, I can be fully present with a patient, forget everything else, and lose myself in the wonderful flow of human connection.

Powerful stuff, certainly, but I believe there's an even higher level of flow to be found in healing, and it's what I've seen my patients achieve when together we create a synchronous, collective flow state of trust and collaboration between doctor and patient. It's like a championship-winning team finding the flow state together at the end of the fourth quarter, but instead of the reward being a trophy, it's a person who has been sick for years finally finding healing and hope. It's a magnificent feeling and the reason I get out of bed every morning; I get to witness miracles every day!

To reach this state of flow in healing, several things must happen, the first of which relates to what Kotler describes when your sense of self vanishes. In healing, this means decoupling from your own story. This may seem counterintuitive because a person's story is so important to finding the root cause of illness, but when it comes time to heal, it's time to draft a new story—a story of healing and wellness, not dysfunction and pain. It starts by letting go of our identity with sickness and recreating a new identity of health and resilience. Healing begins to occur when we begin to think of ourselves in a new way, like when I chose to call myself Sasha, the Warrior Princess, on my chilly walk that morning.

Yes, use your life story and diagnosis to point toward solutions, and use the data from analytical testing on your body to pinpoint specific issues, but then, like an Olympic athlete going for the gold medal, transform your old story by focusing on the *now*—who you are in that present moment, what you are capable of, the ideal version of yourself. Our subconscious is not choosy and will move us toward anything we deeply believe to be true.

Start by writing down and then repeating what you want to become: a redefined, healthier version of *you*. Go grab your journal or a blank sheet of paper. Write it down and then remind yourself frequently of your new identity.

> With time and repetition, your subconscious will have no choice but to act out what you believe to be true about yourself.

Most chronic illness works like this: when you first get sick, you don't even realize it. You were going about your daily life thinking you were healthy but with dysfunction quietly brewing inside and moving you toward a disease state. To heal, the opposite needs to happen. You need to turn yourself around and start walking away from disease, taking small steps in the right direction, even if you still have symptoms or a scary diagnosis. As Earl Nightingale says, "Whatever we plant in our subconscious mind and nourish with repetition and emotion will one day become your reality."

This change in how you talk about yourself encourages healing flow because it redefines who you are on a subconscious level. In addition, there are several common steps that always seem to occur in my patients who find flow and healing in their journey. The following recipe is based on established flow theory, but I've adjusted it to align with my world of medicine:

1. **Get curious.** Ask yourself, "What do I want to do?" "Who do I want to become?" I want to learn to surf. I want to learn to draw. I want to learn to play music. I want to create something new. I want to wake up in the morning and feel good. Curiosity opens the door to all possibility and to healing.

2. **Find meaning and purpose.** Nothing helps with purpose or meaning like believing in a greater force guiding your destiny. Regardless of your spiritual beliefs, finding a purpose and seeking meaning even at the darkest times is crucial. Passion is equally important—finding joy in life will provide you with the energy to get up each day and pursue making a difference in a way that matters to you. Think about what matters most to you and then align your life around these values.

3. **Seek mastery and autonomy.** Study your body, the results provided by testing, and the ways of healing from your diagnosis or symptoms. In my early years as a functional medicine doctor, it wasn't uncommon for my patients to know more about a particular rare illness than I did—and I learned so much from them. Autonomy is important because

you are not relying on someone else for your healing. Instead, you take it on yourself to achieve your dreams and goals for health and prosperity. You may go from feeling like a helpless victim to becoming empowered with the new knowledge and mastery you seek. The moment I started healing from Crohn's disease was when I walked out of my gastroenterologist's office and decided that I could heal myself (autonomy), and in order to do so I needed to embrace a new paradigm of healing (mastery).

Purpose, meaning, and passion, fueled by autonomy and mastery, result in flow. Flow gives us the power to let go of the past and to do what the moment demands. When we reach this state, our body and mind come together, and we are capable of (and receptive to) wondrous miracles, game-winning goals, and impossible healing. In this way, my profession as a healer and my childhood on the farm are not so different. On the farm, we'd walk the beans and remove the weeds that were sucking nutrients away from the crops that we depended on. In functional medicine, we do the same thing in our bodies; we remove the harmful things like fear, anger, toxic relationships, environmental toxins, and processed food, and then we add the healthful parts that bring mind and body together in a biochemical state of flow—nutritional supplements, healthy food, clean air, pure water, resilience, love, joy, hope, and healthy connections.

POWER PLAY

The flow state is closely related to the act of play, which has incredible therapeutic value. We all intuitively know how to harness the power of play as children, but life and conditioning cause us to forget its powerful healing effects. I believe that play is appealing to all ages because by embracing our childlike nature, the resulting flow state opens a portal to our original creativity and intuition. New research from UC Berkeley psychologists suggests that creativity declines as we age, but it doesn't have to be that way.[32]

> By choosing more play, we reignite
> our connection to the natural curiosity
> and creativity of our childhood.

Creativity is also a direct link to the subconscious mind, which holds the keys to every experience, every moment, and every second of our lives and even artifacts from the lives of our ancestors through the genetic material that was handed down to us through transgenerational epigenetic inheritance (how the environment's impact on an individual can affect the traits of future generations).[33]

When I get lost in coloring, dancing, or creative writing, it's an incredible feeling, but more importantly, the endorphins released open the door to deep intuition and more creativity. Connecting to this deep inner wisdom gives us the ability to reprogram our innate fear pathways away from memories of trauma and to instead point the way to healing. This process, sometimes also referred to as "reparenting," was first introduced by Dr. Lucia Capacchione in the 1970s through her art therapy. Reparenting the inner child focuses on making sure we feel value and love that may have been lacking during our childhood. Tapping into our inner child with play and recreation can be one of the strongest medicines we have for healing our psyche and the old toxic trauma we were exposed to long ago.

The type of activity itself doesn't matter. For some it is creative pursuits like dancing, writing, drumming, painting, or coloring, like I do. For others, it might involve a challenging physical activity that requires intense focus or advanced skill, like surfing, skiing, rock climbing, or skydiving. And if you've ever watched a jazz musician improvise, you know that music is another way to achieve the timeless, effortless, creative state of flow.

Much research has been done using neural scanning technology to show how fear, one of the most primal and powerful of emotions, creates ingrained neural pathways in the brain.[34] These pathways become like deeply worn grooves that are easy to fall back into. Anytime your body feels a stressful event, your subconscious opens these well-worn pathways of fear that were created years before and have been reinforced by every stressful event that's happened since. More positive emotions, like love and hope, can also shape these pathways, but once fear has established its route, it is hard to change. But it can be done, and flow-state activities are one of the best ways to rewire those old neural pathways.

This is one reason I love to snow ski. Skiing seems like it's about sliding down a snow-covered mountain, but the most beguiling part of skiing is what happens when fear is transformed into a sense of control, elation, and inspiration. When I point my skis over the edge and see the bird's-eye view of the rolling mountainside below and feel the acceleration, I'm helping my subconscious to rewire my brain. At times, pushing off into deep powder and the unknown may feel scary, but every time I do, I'm teaching my fear to lead me toward joy and pleasure instead. Each time I choose to try something new and challenging despite the fear I feel inside, I gain courage. I begin to trust in my ability to figure things out, releasing the addiction to well-worn fear and trauma pathways that have previously been my default. I create brave new roads to follow, and each time it becomes easier.

Ten Ways to Experience More Flow

1. Choose something you already love to do or try something new.
2. Make it challenging but not too hard. Flow happens right between the two extremes.
3. Clear away other distractions; optimally you should set aside at least four hours for the task.
4. Teach yourself something new—take dancing lessons, learn to surf, go rock climbing, or pick something else that you've always wanted to try.
5. Don't force it. Stop and move on to something different if you are not enjoying yourself.
6. Limit external distractions, silence alerts on your phone, and shut down your Internet browser if you are working on creative writing.
7. Avoid multitasking. Focus only on the one task at hand.
8. Breathe intentionally and let go of any stress; surrender to the process.
9. Listen to music that enhances flow. I like to use Focus@Will for alpha wave–inducing music while I am working creatively.
10. Use a PEMF mat (I like HigherDose) or red light therapy (Sauna Space or VieLight for the brain) to jump-start the process.

For more information on flow state inducers, visit www.ReadUnexpected.com/Resources.

PATIENT HAS THE ANSWERS

I quickly found myself with the daunting task of helping patients with incredibly complex and challenging health conditions. In Peoria, I'd used holistic methods to offer additional healing opportunities for patients who were already being supported by the traditional allo-pathic medical system. In my new practice, I started seeing many people for whom the medical system had completely failed.

Consider Nancy, who came to see me after she had been subjected to a list of treatments and diagnoses that defy imagination. She had cognitive issues, had seen an eye doctor for blurry vision, had been given a brain scan to rule out multiple sclerosis, and was prescribed medication for migraines that were so bad she would often vomit the migraine medicine before it had a chance to take effect. Multiple rheumatologists had given her their best shot, including expensive immune-modulating injections after she was diagnosed with psoriatic arthritis. One doctor simply wrote the diagnosis of depression on her record even though she had never mentioned any complaints related to her mood.

"When I was twenty-six, they told me I lived in the body of an eighty-year-old," she said. "I suppose that's enough to make anyone depressed."

A sports medicine doctor said her health issues were because of poor form when running. A dermatologist prescribed powerful steroid cream for her psoriasis. A holistic doctor gave her a food intolerance test, and she left with a list of only eight foods she could eat.

"I was taking pills around the clock for ten years," she said. "One doctor would put me on track and tell me to march, so I'd march. Then another doctor would put me on another track and tell me to march, so I'd march. I was given a colonoscopy and other invasive treatments that I didn't need, and none of it helped me to feel better."

As with so many of my patients, Nancy's issues went way back. In high school she had been a competitive gymnast and runner but had to forfeit the state championship due to excruciating pain. She tried acupuncture and other alternative therapies, but nothing worked.

In college she suffered from psoriasis to such a degree that rashes covered 50 percent of her body and she had installed a UV treatment bed in student housing to help with her skin issues.

"It was really weird for my roommates," she said. "It looked like a tanning bed, and they were always having to explain that it was for therapy, not vanity."

Upon reading her medical history, I knew we were going to have to do a comprehensive work-up, so on her very first appointment, we drew thirty-two vials of blood for a wide variety of tests. We waited for the results, which would allow us to develop a treatment plan based on a foundation of analytical data. We found several infections, positive genetics for celiac disease, evidence of severe intestinal permeability, dangerously elevated inflammatory markers in the blood, and many food intolerances.

The previous years of medications had destroyed the integrity of Nancy's gut, and I knew we had to work on healing her gut first. She improved dramatically with the gut treatment, but some issues persisted, so I ordered western blot and PCR testing for a battery of infectious diseases, including tick-borne infections. Thanks to our rapidly warming world, ticks are expanding their range, and the incidence of vector illnesses like Lyme disease and other coinfections are increasing enormously; the US EPA reports that Lyme prevalence per capita doubled between 1991 and 2018, with most experts agreeing that the actual number of infections is far higher than what's reported.[35] Sure enough, Nancy tested positive for an infection called Bartonella, or "cat scratch disease." She took triple intracellular antibiotics to target the bacteria in separate phases of its life cycle, and we also added probiotics and immunoglobulins to protect her microbiome from the negative impact of the antibiotics.

What Is Neuroplasticity?

"Our brain's adaptability to respond to input from our internal and external environment is called neuroplasticity. It continues from conception throughout our life until the minute we die. Knowing that our brain and nervous system have this magnificent built-in change capacity engenders endless hope. How wonderful to know that we have a brain that keeps reimagining its potential as we reimagine ours!"

ILENE NAOMI RUSK, PhD
DIRECTOR, HEALTHY BRAIN PROGRAM
THE BRAIN + BEHAVIOR CLINIC

Dr. Jill's Tips for Enhancing Neuroplasticity
1. Commit to reading every day
2. Drive a different route to work
3. Do something you've always done in a brand-new way
4. Challenge yourself to word puzzles every morning
5. Travel and explore unfamiliar places and diverse cultures
6. Learn a new skill, try a new sport, get creative, color!
7. Teach yourself a new language or new musical instrument

By enlisting flow and changing our mindset, we can rewire our brain in a very real way that makes us more resilient through a phenomenon called neuroplasticity.

Today, Nancy says she's ninety percent healed, but she's still on a journey. The massive transformation she has already seen in her health has provided a great deal of motivation to keep going. When she is talking with other parents at a school event and the subject of mysterious symptoms comes up, she never misses the opportunity to share her optimism.

She says, "They are so surprised when I tell them how I was so sick for much of my life. They say, 'You? You are the pinnacle of health!'"

Nancy, like me, is still improving her health every day, but she has embraced the journey, as she puts it, as a "life quest." Interestingly, most successful patients look at health this way; they don't really see themselves as healed as much as they view healing as a way of life. The more I learn about how the brain responds to strong emotional messages, like hope and its darker cousin, fear, I can understand how these patients are not just being optimistic but are physically transforming their brains to support healing. That's neuroplasticity.

HEALING OUR GAME

After a few years in Colorado, my reputation as a functional medicine expert spread, and other doctors began seeking me out as a consultant. I quickly realized that functional medicine isn't just for helping people who are sick; it can also be used to optimize performance, improve vitality with age, and increase quality of life at any age. In the post-pandemic world, as we heal from the worst health crisis in a century, this approach to health is proving to be more important than ever.

When Dr. Chad Prusmack, an Ivy League–educated physician and the official neurosurgeon for the Denver Broncos and the US Olympic teams, first emailed me to ask for help, I was quick to call him back. I was floored that he was asking for my expertise and was delighted to help functional medicine expand into new arenas. He hired me to teach him the principles of functional medicine as he developed the Resilience Code, a program designed to integrate the bio-investigative technology I use in my clinic with a world-class training facility. While I have met many neurosurgeons, Dr. Prusmack defies all stereotypes. Somehow he managed to get through a brutal amount of training in one of the most competitive fields of medicine and maintain one of the deepest hearts of compassion I have ever seen.

When a member joins the Resilience Code—be it an athlete, entrepreneur, or anyone interested in increasing their performance—they are given a series of tests with three clear goals: to measure improvement, track vitality, and fight disease. Kinetic testing includes 3D movement evaluation, skeletal motion and gait analysis, VO2 and lactate testing, and sports-specific testing, including mobility, relative strength, power, and endurance. Biological testing includes bone density, nutrition, food sensitivity, lipids, vitals, and 3D body scanning. Heart testing includes medical history evaluation, stress echocardiogram, and ultrasound. Cancer resistance testing includes genetics, blood biomarker, microbiome, and hematology. Everyone is given a monitor that will collect physiological data around the clock. And that's just the beginning.

He then uses this baseline to develop a "resilience code" that clearly explains the individual's strengths, weaknesses, and unique biology. Working with a team of trainers and nutritionists, Dr. Prusmack develops a training program based on an individual's data. Then, over time, they can track their progress with real data and adjust their code accordingly.

Dr. Prusmack was a quick study, and I helped him to understand how to both intuitively and analytically use the data from an individual's test results to paint a picture of their health that they could use to help them make lifestyle decisions. He went on to add functional medicine certification to his neurosurgeon credentials, and his facility grew into one of the most advanced performance health centers in the world. His team of physical therapists, personal trainers, massage therapists, sports psychologists, and functional medicine doctors work together to interpret their clients' data to give the center's members the optimal chance of living their healthiest lives possible.

If everyone had access to a facility like the Resilience Code, we could cut the prevalence of lifestyle disease by an enormous amount. The club itself consists of forty thousand square feet of the most advanced therapy and training equipment ever designed, including antigravity and proprioception machines, a UV sauna, sequential hot and cold tubs, pressure suits for lymphatic stimulation, an intravenous nutrient room complete with overstuffed chairs big enough to hold three-hundred-pound linebackers and equipped with IV delivery systems, a full muscle-activation therapy lab, and even a mixed martial arts fighting cage.

Half of the Resilience Code members are people looking for life improvement, and the other half are professional athletes. Long-term members, especially those who end up being sick or injured in any way during their time as members, collect data, such as daily vital signs, to help them optimize their healing. As Dr. Prusmack says, "This is the way to change health care; we use the data to make you the expert."

While helping Dr. Prusmack, I realized that what he was offering his clients was exactly what I had been doing for myself for decades. Teaching patients how to optimize performance by tuning in to science and intuition was a powerful way to achieve better physical and mental health each day, defying expectations of declining health at any age. Clearly, I wasn't the only physician connecting the flow state of athletes to the flow state of healing.

Travel Tips for Optimal Performance

Travel often entails a dose of toxicity: exposure to cleaning products in hotels, polluted air, stress, and less-than-optimal food choices.

Here are some simple tips to travel well:

Planning:

- Give yourself extra time getting to the airport and making connections. A tight travel schedule adds pointless stress.
- Research healthy grocery options and allergen-friendly restaurants where you are traveling. (Try apps like Find Me Gluten Free.)
- Pack specialty items you may not be able to purchase at your destination. For me, this includes protein bars, organic coffee, and grain-free granola.
- Optimize sleep. Use melatonin to optimize your circadian rhythm in the days leading up to your trip if you are traveling across time zones.

In Flight:

- Pack a stainless-steel water bottle with integrated filter straw so you can filter tap water easily. I like the Clearly Filtered water bottle.
- Use noise-canceling headphones in transit.
- Wear blue-blockers on the plane to avoid ambient light entering the peripheral retina.
- Take an immune-boosting dose of vitamin D3.

- Travel with a stash of you-friendly food. Don't rely on airports, as they rarely have healthy options. (I pack grain-free bars, chopped-up vegetables like red bell peppers, organic berries, and dark chocolate.)

Hotels:
- Look for hypoallergenic rooms with medical-grade air purification systems. Some chains give guests a hypo-allergic option when booking their room.
- Ask that no fragrances or toxic chemicals be used for cleaning your room.
- Ask for a mini fridge in your room so you can store and prepare clean food and any medications.
- Have a service like Instacart or Amazon Whole Foods deliver food to your room upon arrival.
- Ask for a room with windows that open to the outside so you can dilute the cleaning chemicals or air pollut-ants upon arrival by opening windows.
- Bring your own organic mycotoxin-free coffee and travel French press to make your own brew toxin-free in your room. I also travel with a collapsible silicone hot pot for easy access to hot water for tea or coffee.

For more of my favorite products, visit www.Read Unexpected.com/Resources.

CLEAN AIR, CLEAN WATER, CLEAN FOOD

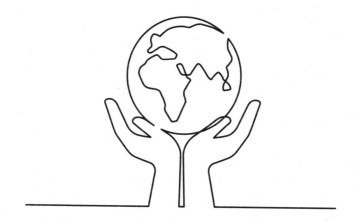

When it comes to overcoming complex and chronic health problems, the most critical therapy isn't complex treatment protocols or trendy detoxification plans. Instead, it always starts with three fundamentals: clean air, clean water, and clean food. These factors are so significant that it almost makes my job easy. Even short-term exposure to elevated levels of small particulates in the air is associated with an increase in heart attacks.[36] In my view, this statistic is encouraging; it means that we can reduce the risk of heart attack by simply breathing clean air! In fact, one of my greatest teachers, the late Dr. Walter Crinnion, would say that 80 percent of our environmental toxic exposure comes from the air we breathe!

When my patients make a concerted effort to breathe unpolluted air; to eat food that is free of chemicals, pesticides, and additives; and to drink pure, filtered, or natural spring water, their health invariably improves. Likewise, no amount of complex detoxification protocols will take away the need for choosing to put clean inputs into our body.

My bout with cancer and the potential connections with growing up on a farm inspired many conversations with my dad and brothers. Once they considered the dangers, they decided to change many of their farming practices. Of course, being experienced farmers and knowing the fickle nature of their business, they wanted to be careful not to destroy their livelihood in the process. At that time, nobody in their region grew organically, and virtually everyone was using genetically modified crops. The other farmers they talked to laughed at them when they mentioned the idea of organic farming.

But they also could see that if they were careful in how they converted to a cleaner way of farming, there would also be greater premium or value in producing healthier food in a less environmentally damaging way. They started small and converted some of their acreage to non-GMO and a smaller section to organic. Then, as farmers do, they waited for proof of life. Sure enough, the organic and non-GMO crops grew beautifully. It required a change in the way they farmed, and they spent money on hired help to pull weeds instead of on herbicides. But it wasn't until after the harvest and the food was sold to the market that the final score was tallied.

The results were amazing. Not only did cleaner farming produce better food; the organic and non-GMO products were better business. Over the next couple of seasons, they converted the entire operation to non-GMO and increased the portion of their farm that was producing certified organic crops. My dad says, "Jill was right: the farm was healthier, the food we grew was better, and, in the end, we are more profitable."

> When teaching about the power of
> functional medicine, I always start with,
> "Clean air, clean water, clean food."

Patients are also surprised to hear that some of the most important principles in healing didn't involve complex protocols but simply choosing to be more aware of what they put in their bodies. I researched water-filtration systems and air purifiers and started recommending certain ones with high-quality HEPA and VOC filters or encouraged them to make the move to a place with cleaner air if possible. We run multiple high-quality air filters in the office, and many patients would comment on how clean the air felt when they came to visit. Each patient leaves with instructions on how to minimize pesticide exposure; avoid high-mercury foods; purchase local and organic, non-GMO food when possible; avoid all refined and processed foods; and install a water-filtration system to provide the most basic essential, clean water. As the world grows more polluted and toxins prevail, the value of taking even small steps to reduce toxic load makes a huge difference. I thought I knew everything there was to know about toxicity, but the next life lesson would blow this notion to shreds.

Living Well in a Toxic World

Healing doesn't have to be complicated: work less, play more, chase flow, embrace gratitude, and share love. Here are my top tips for living well in a toxic world.

1. Clean Air

- Equip your home with high-quality HEPA filtration systems that contain a filter for volatile organic compounds (VOCs). I like Austin Air and AirDoctor.
- Replace your furnace filter every three months with a high-quality filter rated MERV 7 or greater.
- Identify and eliminate common sources of off-gassing in your home, like new carpet, laminate cabinets, or flooring or upholstered furniture and mattresses, which often contain flame retardants.
- Switch from natural gas appliances to electric when possible.
- Avoid using artificial air freshener products in your home.

2. Clean Water

- Drink filtered, spring, or glass bottled mineral water.
- Install a reverse osmosis whole-house water filtration system or countertop filtration system like Berkey water or use a Clearly Filtered pitcher.

3. Clean Food

- Choose organic, pesticide- and chemical-free, locally grown, non-GMO produce and adhere to a

Mediterranean-style, primarily plant-based, gluten-free diet.
- Avoid excess plastics and packaging when choosing food at the supermarket.

4. Clean Mind

- Work through personal trauma with somatic-based therapies, like eye movement desensitization and reprocessing (EMDR), neurolinguistic programming (NLP), Emotional Freedom Technique (EFT), Internal Family Systems Therapy (IFS) and others.
- Relieve stress by hiking in nature, listening to binaural beats, and practicing heart rate variability training or other things that calm an overactive nervous system.
- Optimize your relationships by engaging a therapist who understands attachment theory and how it impacts you and/or your partner.

5. Clean Body

- Incorporate sweating through exercise or infrared sauna.
- Support lymphatic drainage with dry brushing, hydrotherapy, and Epsom salt baths.
- Keep your gut happy with spore probiotics and fibers, like psyllium or citrus pectin, and support digestion with bitters and digestive enzymes.

For more of my favorite products, visit www.ReadUnexpected.com/Resources.

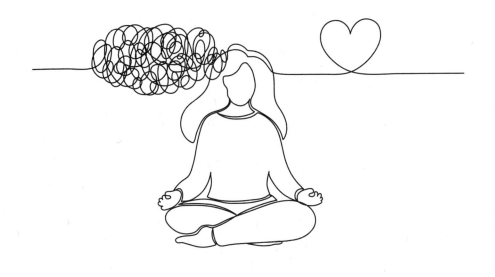

CHAPTER 6

How to Transform Toxicity

In some ways suffering ceases to be suffering at the moment
it finds a meaning, such as the meaning of a sacrifice.
—Viktor E. Frankl, author of
Man's Search for Meaning

THE THOUSAND-YEAR FLOOD

The soft, rhythmic beat of the windshield wipers lulled me into a reverie that morning. The heavy clouds and steady rain that I drove through on the way to my clinic on September 11, 2013, were a refreshing change from a sizzling dry summer and seemed a fitting memorial to the attacks on New York and the first day of my chemotherapy for breast cancer—both twelve years earlier to the day. At first it didn't seem like dangerous rain. It was hardly a downpour compared with the typical thunderstorms that built over the high peaks of the Continental Divide. These storms typically pelted the towns along the Front Range with hailstones the size of golf balls and inches of rain. They would blow past an hour later, leaving blue skies, rainbows, and a refreshing smell from the negative ions left behind. But unlike a typical summer thunderstorm, this time the rain didn't stop.

The dozen years that had passed since the fateful call with Dr. Smith had been a dream come true. If anyone asked Aaron or I how our relationship was, both of us would have said, "Just perfect." We traveled together, we were living a stone's throw from the Rocky Mountains, and we skied together nearly every Friday. When I was a little girl, my Midwestern father had the insight to take his entire family of five children to the Rockies on a shoestring budget every winter until we fell in love with the adventurous winter sport. Sporting Carhartt's mismatched mittens, hand-me-down ski coats, and a Midwestern enthusiasm, we arrived early to the chair lift to make "first tracks" and skied until the last run at 4 p.m., squeezing every moment out of our annual ski week.

Our wedding vows had an unspoken clause: Aaron had to learn to ski. To his credit, he was a good sport although I was a terrible teacher. When he unloaded from the chair lift for the first time, legs wobbling like a toddler's first steps, my only advice was, "Just swish your butt." Then I took off down the mountain before he could blink, leaving him with no choice but to follow or get left behind. I do recall wondering if the tender early days of our marriage would withstand these first ski "lessons." But he learned to ski quickly. Skiing and our love of the mountains were a big part of our decision to move to Colorado.

After struggling with illness and overwhelming workload through my twenties and early thirties, I was finally enjoying the best health of my life. Moving away from the farm chemicals, moldy corn, and soybean dust that had plagued my youth and finding unconditional acceptance in a free-spirited, health-minded community had bolstered my strength and confidence. I felt for the first time in my life that I had found my "tribe" and aligned with like-minded, health-conscious friends and neighbors. I almost forgot how I had once felt so out of place growing up in my hometown of Roanoke, Illinois. That year I ran the BOLDERBoulder 10K race in a competitive time and was hiking up mountains all summer and skiing down them all winter. I didn't have a formal business plan, but my vision of creating a functional medicine practice where my ulti-mate dream—loving patients and changing lives—was becoming reality. I shared a quaint 1970s oak-trimmed office with Dr. Rountree and had a highly dedicated office staff who shared my vision and helped make it happen by serving up hope one patient at a time. Driving through a September rainstorm on the way to the office got me thinking about that difficult day twelve years earlier when I had stared my own mortality in the face, but life had been so good for me in recent years. The rain didn't dampen my spirits in the slightest.

By the evening of the following day, Boulder had received as much precipitation as it usually sees in an entire year, and the governor had declared a federal emergency in fourteen counties. Six people were confirmed dead and another thousand were missing. Roads were obliterated as the steep-sided canyons cutting into the foothills were reshaped by what was effectively a seven-thousand-foot waterfall pouring off the Continental Divide. Residents scrambled to escape the raging waters, and thanks to experienced rescue teams, the thousand missing people all turned up alive.

The National Oceanic and Atmospheric Association declared the storm a thousand-year event, and the price tag on the damage was estimated at a billion dollars. But that didn't even include the indirect costs, like the catastrophic impact that a little flood damage to my office building would have on my practice, my health, and even my marriage. Just as two low pressure systems collide to form extreme storms, a combination of factors (environmental, emotional, and relational) were about to collide with a destructive synergy and shatter my life in ways that would make cancer and Crohn's seem little more than a sprained ankle.

IN-TO-ME-SEE

As the floodwaters receded, Aaron was off in Nashville for weeks at a time, working as artistic director and manager for his musician cousin and best friend since childhood, Rory Feek, and Rory's wife, Joey. Aaron's constant travel seemed like a stable balance to my own demanding schedule, at least at first.

My clinic had a yearlong wait list, and I was speaking at medical conferences around the world. Aaron and I didn't take as much time to go skiing together, and any travel we did together usually dovetailed with a conference of mine. But that's life, right?

Wrong.

Living in the mountains of Colorado felt like a vacation destination, so we hadn't been on a real vacation together in years. A relationship as solid as ours didn't need such niceties as relaxing weekends of frolic or vacations without work, right?

Wrong.

After getting through cancer, Aaron and I could handle anything, right?

Wrong.

When Aaron took the job in Nashville, we decided that he would be gone for no more than a week each month and that we would stay connected by phone or video calls while he traveled. It wasn't long before his absences extended far beyond our one-week agreement. Something deep inside me was stirring, a feeling I associated with weakness and covered over with a hard shell of self-reliance and the lie I told myself, sometimes out loud: "I am just fine, thank you!"

It was loneliness.

We had long lived by an unspoken rule, one that seemed like a clever idea on the surface: "You take care of you, and I'll take care of me." We were so independent that we rarely even ate meals together. I would go to the fridge and make a leafy green salad with walnuts, strawberries, and organic chicken, while he would grab takeout on his way home. As a result, for much of our marriage we lived parallel lives, but in true intimacy, we sorely lacked. I now realize that while we thought we were deeply connected; we were busy denying our own needs and avoiding true vulnerability. We were particularly good at pretending we were okay and unskilled at asking for what we needed from each other. Someone once said that intimacy is "in-to-me-see," a play on pronunciation filled with wisdom. But we didn't get it. Our play was a farce, and we walked on stage playing the parts of two eternal optimists who had wonderful adventures and incredible intellectual conversations, but I don't think we ever allowed ourselves to be truly vulnerable with each other.

We told everyone that our independence made us stronger. In our minds we were an unstoppable powerhouse of ideas and success, but in our hearts, we were both suffering from toxic stress and a lack of support. Further sealing our fate, we hadn't developed an awareness of our emotional health, our needs, or how to be honest with each other, which might have allowed us to identify the problem before it spiraled out of control. Laughing when we felt like crying was the armor we both bravely wore, at least in front of each other. It seemed to us like the perfect recipe for marital bliss. Avoiding conflict should make a marriage better, right?

Wrong again.

This overly optimistic self-denial approach to life went far deeper than my marriage. It started all the way back in my childhood when I didn't tell my parents I really needed some quiet time reading rather than taking on the massive responsibilities of the household chores and caring for my younger siblings.

> I was joyful Jill, the eternal optimist
> and grandmaster at the game of
> suppressing my true feelings, and
> I had a reputation to maintain.

During chemotherapy there were times I could only lie in bed, curled in a miserable ball, but I never complained. I would make jokes about being glabrous instead of telling the truth that I was bald and ashamed of how I looked. I became so good at faking it. I remember standing naked and alone in my bedroom, sobbing while I looked in the mirror at my thin frame, cue-ball head, and left breast ravaged by angry scars. I felt utterly alone and completely unworthy of love. How could anyone possibly love this tattered, hairless, battle-scarred girl? But after crying my eyes out, I washed my face, put on a little mascara and some tinted moisturizer to hide the tear tracks on my cheeks, donned my platinum blond wig, and went out to greet Aaron with a cheerful smile and asked sweetly, "What would you like for dinner, honey?"

Is it any wonder I married a man who also preferred to avoid conflict and difficult conversations? We were both so strong in suppressing our emotions that we might have preserved our illusions of perfection for many more years if it weren't for a movie in Virginia, some arachnids, and microscopic toxins from the thousand-year flood.

JOSEPHINE

Joey and Rory captured the world's attention, first as a talented wife-and-husband musical act and then through Rory's online journal of Joey's struggle with cervical cancer that eventually claimed her life. Joey and I were fast friends, close in age and sharing a common upbringing in the Midwestern farm country, with strong faith and a devotion to a very practical, selfless, nurturing motherhood of stepchildren. During visits to their farmhouse in Tennessee, after the dinner dishes were cleared off the table and the two of us were left sitting together, we had many conversations the likes of which I don't think either of us had before.

One evening, Joey said quietly, "Jill, Rory wants another baby more than anything. Didn't you ever want children of your own?"

I remember looking at her beautiful, honest face and then saying, "The truth is, I never really had that dream of wedding dresses and babies in high school like so many of my friends. I suppose instead I nurtured a passion for helping people heal, and I knew I couldn't pour all my heart into both service and motherhood. Between the instant family after marrying Aaron (who had three children from a previous marriage) and getting breast cancer in my twenties, I think God answered the question for me."

"Such a lovely perspective, Jill." She smiled and squeezed my hand.

I could relate to the pressure she felt. Being raised in a conservative Midwestern community but not having the desire to bear children was inconceivable. My siblings all have kids, and most of my childhood friends had married and had babies by the time they turned twenty-five. In that culture, a woman's place was in the home taking care of the children, not in medical school or traveling the

world keynoting on stages. I realize now that my willingness to marry
a man with three stepchildren had something to do with the fact that
it got me off the hook for the expectation of starting my own family.
But my own lack of maternal desire always felt like a dirty secret. I
told her I dreamed of becoming a healer and inspiring people, not
having babies. Joey was the first person with whom I ever shared this
deep secret, and doing so was an enormous weight off my chest.

It wasn't long before Joey became pregnant and they had a beautiful baby girl, named Indiana, who brought great joy into their lives.
But after giving birth, she lost an incredible amount of blood, surviving
only after a transfusion to restore the blood loss. She was diagnosed
with cervical cancer shortly after the birth of Indiana. Cancer was a
darker common thread intertwining our lives.

Joey loved her precious baby girl as much as I have ever seen a
mother love a baby. Talk about unexpected miracles—giving birth to
her darling baby girl changed Joey in the deepest sense; she became
the most amazing mother I have ever seen. During the sweetest part
of Joey and Rory's lives, celebrating her cancer being in remission,
doting on their new baby girl, and enjoying a successful career, Aaron
and Rory decided to make a movie called *Josephine*. Inspired by letters
he found when he bought a 150-year-old farmhouse, Rory penned a
story about the wife of a Civil War soldier who poses as a man so she
can enlist in the army and fight her way across the country to find her
missing husband. Aaron and Rory worked together to write the script
and then cast, shoot, and produce the film. It was a dream come true
for both but also a stressful nightmare of overwhelming magnitude.
After filming all day, Aaron and Rory would barely have time to take
a shower; pull the creepy, blood-sucking ticks off their skin that had
found their way into their clothes while shooting scenes in the thick
Virginia forest; choke down some food; and then work deep into the
night planning the next day's production. Aaron was gone for months

at a time. He poured his heart and soul into making the movie, but it left little time or energy for anything else, including our marriage.

Sometimes while he was away, we talked on the phone and Aaron would share bits and pieces of the daily drama. I would also share my day-to-day experiences but rarely told him how much I was struggling inside too. Expressing my own exhaustion and overwhelm may have helped him to understand, but I had never learned to speak the language of expressing my true feelings. Turns out, he hadn't learned it either. We were both dying inside and yet neither of us knew how to express it.

ELEPHANT ANKLES

The red, scaly, peeling skin around my eyes and my swollen grandma-like ankles should have clued me in, but I didn't really understand that something was wrong until I had to stop to catch my breath while climbing the stairs to my second-floor office. I also noticed that while typing or speaking, sometimes names or other words would come out wrong. My complex thinking, like solving difficult medical problems and designing treatment plans, was still completely intact. It was bizarre; I could quickly see clues leading to a diagnosis in a 150-page medical history but then forget the name of the patient.

Knowing that we had just endured a devastating flood and that difficulty finding words is a hallmark of mold-related illness, I intuitively knew what was happening. As the planet warms, droughts have plagued many areas, but the occurrence of heavy rainfall has increased in others, including the United States.[37] This means more buildings are being damaged in ways that allow for mold growth, and clinics like mine are seeing an incredible increase in the number of patients with mold toxicity and other issues that are closely related to the changing environment.

But just as I often saw with my patients, even as I considered the likelihood that my office was infested with mold, I remained in denial for several months. If I was sick from mold toxicity, healing was going to be life-altering, and I wasn't mentally prepared for the dramatic changes that would be needed. Exacerbating the problem tremendously, mold toxicity has a sneaky way of amplifying overwhelm and taking away insight. Mold toxins are devious little gremlins that not only make you sick but also make it much harder to do the very thing that will make you better. Can you imagine what would happen if dehydration prevented you from feeling thirsty?

My symptoms worsened by the day, and I began to feel that daunting déjà vu from my past brushes with severe illness: first, I had to get past denial; second, I knew that there had to be solutions, and I was determined to find them once again; and third, I knew these lessons would become the basis for helping others get through the utter despair of environmental illness and regain their health in the future. I would have never chosen to be "the mold expert," as I've been referred to in the years since, but "I didn't choose mold; it chose me." Or as my Jewish friend, Dr. Rusk, told me one morning while hiking, "Jill, God knew you had the chutzpah to handle this crazy mold adventure with grace and resilience."

The troublemakers in mold are called mycotoxins, chemical compounds produced by some molds that are released into the air we breathe, which can wreak havoc on the body. Mycotoxins are tiny, as small as 0.1 microns in size, about the same size as the coronavirus that caused the pandemic, half the size of the average bacteria and a thousand times smaller than the width of a human hair. Like other environmental toxins, including pesticides, toxic food additives, or air pollution, dealing with mycotoxins from a mold growing in the home or workplace is a little like trying to keep a fish tank algae-free without ever washing it. I was literally swimming in a toxic soup, breathing in the mycotoxins with every breath I took.

TOXIC LOAD + INFECTIOUS BURDEN

I believe most of my patients with complex and chronic illness have some combination of toxic load and infectious burden. This combination weakens the immune system and further leads to inflammation and autoimmunity. Doctors like me who treat complex environmental illnesses often find both mold-related illness (a toxin) and infectious diseases, like tick-borne illness or viruses like Epstein-Barr or cytomegalovirus (infections), in the same patient. I believe that if we tested ten thousand people off the street, we would find that many of them would test positive for antibodies to tick-borne infections like Lyme disease, sometimes from a tick bite decades earlier, but few would be symptomatic, need treatment, or even know they had been infected. When our immune system is strong and healthy, we don't have the symptoms of these low-virulence infections. Infections like Ebola virus are high virulence, meaning they cause death within days. Tick-borne infections like Borrelia burgdorferi and viruses like Epstein Barr, while more common, are also low virulence and cause little harm in the context of a strong, healthy immune system.

However, molds like Chaetomium or Stachybotrys produce known immune-suppressive mycotoxins, like mycophenolic acid, which is the main ingredient in immunosuppressive drugs like myco-phenolate mofetil, prescribed for those receiving organ transplants. When a patient is living in a moldy environment, the exposure to mycotoxins naturally weakens the immune system. This exposure then wrecks their body's ability to keep old infections in check, ones that were previously not causing symptoms. Suddenly they present with increased joint pain, fatigue, and cognitive disturbances, which are hallmarks of the reactivation of these old infections due to the immune-suppressive effects of mold.

Signs and Symptoms of Mold Exposure

Many patients are unaware that their home or workplace could be the breeding ground for their symptoms. In fact, it's estimated that indoor pollutants, including toxic mold, are at a concentration of two to five times higher than that of the pollutants found outdoors and contribute to more than 50 percent of patients' illnesses. By far the most common health issue caused by mold is allergy.

Mold-related allergic reactions include:

- coughing
- wheezing
- red, itchy, and watery eyes
- runny nose
- rash

If you're someone who already has chronic or seasonal allergies or suffers from a respiratory condition such as asthma or COPD (Chronic Obstructive Pulmonary Disease), your allergic reaction to mold may be much more significant.

These worsened allergic symptoms can cause:

- persistent coughing
- headaches
- difficulty breathing
- sinus inflammation
- fatigue and lethargy
- frequent illness/weakened immune system

In cases of long-term toxic mold exposure, this may lead to more serious symptoms such as:

- fatigue and weakness
- frequent headaches, light sensitivity
- poor memory, confusion, difficulty concentrating
- difficulty with word finding
- morning stiffness, joint pain
- muscle cramping
- unusual skin sensations
- tingling and numbness in your hands and feet
- shortness of breath
- sinus pressure/congestion
- chronic dry cough
- appetite swings, body temperature dysregulation
- unexplained weight loss or weight gain
- increased in urinary frequency and thirst
- red eyes, blurry vision, night sweats
- mood swings, irritability, depression, anxiety, insomnia
- sharp "ice pick"-like pains
- abdominal pain, diarrhea, gas, bloating
- hair loss
- metallic taste in mouth
- static shocks
- dizziness, lightheadedness

Nearly every one of my confirmed mold toxicity patients shows signs and symptoms of a weakened immune system. If they had been infected by borrelia, bartonella, babesia, or other tick-borne infections in the past, this exposure to mold can lower the bar of their immune system to the point that old infection rears its ugly head. As a result, it is extremely common for both toxic exposures, like mold, and infectious burden, like tick-borne infections or reactivated old viruses, to appear in the same patient and cause a set of symptoms that encompasses many systems, often confusing a clinician who is not trained in the complexity of environmental toxicity or functional medicine.

I hear this story all the time: "I have hiked and camped in the woods for years and was pulling ticks off of me all the time, but I never had a problem, never had symptoms. Then we moved to a new house with water damage, and I started getting sick with symptoms of joint pain, brain fog, and severe fatigue. I thought I was just getting older." The good news is that the opposite is also true. When we identify and lower the toxic load, our immune system has more bandwidth to handle other infections and other assaults on the body, and these patients can once again experience optimal health and vitality. The first step, however, is identifying the source of mold exposure and getting out!

THE RANCH HAND'S DAUGHTER

While I had seen quite a few patients with mycotoxin illness prior to my own exposure, I truly had no idea the extent of physical suffering and mental anguish they were going through until I experienced it myself. And I was lucky. I discovered the source of the danger and was able to remove myself from the moldy environment and begin repairing my system within a period of months. One of my patients, Sara, tells what is, unfortunately, a much more common mycotoxin illness story that spans decades.

"I was pretty much always sick," Sara said, looking back on her childhood.

Sara grew up in a small ranching community in Montana. Her dad was a ranch hand, and they moved frequently between jobs. Old linoleum, water damage, and musty carpet were standard features in the ranch hand's house. When her dad got a new job, her parents

What to Do if You Suspect Mold-Related Illness

If you are afraid to consider that mold toxicity might be contributing to your symptoms, you are not alone. Here is my step-by-step approach to determine if mold may be part of the problem.

- Did the onset of symptoms relate to a change in environment or a new home or workplace?
- Have you had water damage of any kind in your home or workplace.
- Do online visual contrast testing to screen for biotoxin exposure.
    - Free VCS testing site (https://www.vcstest.com)
    - Surviving mold (https://www.survivingmold.com)
- Make a list of your symptoms. Do they fit with mold-related illness? See the symptom in "Signs and Symptoms of Mold Exposure" on page 162.
- Test your body (your doctor may need to order these tests)
    - Check inflammatory markers in your blood (TGF beta, MMP-9, MSH, VEGF, ADH, osmolality, copeptin, C3a, and C4a)
    - Urinary mycotoxin testing: Real Time Labs, Great Plains, and Vibrant
    - Nasal cultures for bacteria (MARCoNs) and fungus or mold
    - Urinary organic acid testing
    - Rule out MCAS (mast cell activation syndrome)

- Test your home
    - o Start with ordering qPCR testing for your home and workplace. Test kits can be ordered from Mycometrics or EnviroBiomics.
    - o Hire a qualified inspector or Indoor Environmental Professional (IEP) to identify the source of mold in your home.
    For referrals to trained professionals, visit the websites of the International Society for Environmentally Acquired Illness (ISEAI), the Building Biology Institute, or the American Council for Accredited Certification (ACAC).
    - o Get a remediation expert to give you an estimate to repair or correct the issue.
- Find a qualified mold-literate physician to help you create a healing plan. You can search for providers in your area on the ISEAI website.
- For more information watch my interviews with experts on mold and MCAS on my YouTube Channel.
- Start detoxing! Learn more at https://molddetoxbox.com and see the section "Steps to Heal from Mold-Related Illness" on page 184.

bought a house and, taking a leap of faith based on an intuitive sense that something in the old building materials was bothering their daughter, took out a loan and rebuilt the home's interior. It worked. Sara felt better.

"I was like a new kid!" she says.

But for her, the pendulum between health and sickness didn't stop there. In high school, her health hit a new low; her stomach troubles worsened, and she was diagnosed with irritable bowel syndrome (IBS). While the sickness was debilitating, that wasn't the part she hated the most. "The worst was missing school and activities and being at home vomiting and not knowing why," she said. I suspect she had been unwittingly exposed to a common mycotoxin aptly, but unpleasantly, named vomitoxin, which is found in a mold called Fusarium that grows on grains.

Like so many of us who have overcome health challenges, Sara's instinct to solve problems is strong, and with no education on the matter she started trying to figure out what made her sick. Her efforts helped immensely, but in college she had random bouts of intestinal issues like food poisoning. She visited more doctors, but they just said, "It must be your IBS."

After college, she married and started a family. But pregnancy was difficult, with excessive vomiting and difficult labor. Her second pregnancy was even worse, and the list of foods she could tolerate shrank to four items.

But her third pregnancy made the others seem like holidays by comparison. She was in bed the entire nine months. Sara came to see me after her symptoms worsened to include depression, severe fatigue, and leg pain she described as being like trying to sprint as fast as possible when horribly out of shape. As is so common with my patients, Sara confided in me that she had been told by multiple doctors to stop asking questions, to stop researching and take the medication they prescribed. As usual, I took the opposite approach and told her that her research was welcome and that she could ask me as many questions as she wanted.

We had just started making progress healing her gut, and her bouts with depression and pain were lessening, when her kids started having strange issues. Her youngest child began wetting the bed, and another started having chronic nosebleeds and sleepwalking. When she told me this, my intuition screamed, "Mycotoxins!"

I said, "I think you may have mold in your house."

Steps You Can Take to Prevent Mold Growth

As you read earlier, it's impossible to prevent all mold growth since spores are always floating in the air. However, here are some steps you can take to discourage future growth:

- Control the moisture by investing in a dehumidifier and keep humidity levels under 50 percent.
- Dry wet spots immediately.
- Keep areas prone to mold growth cleaned, disinfected, and dry.
- Have your HVAC professionally cleaned every year.
- Fix leaks immediately. If there is water damage under a sink, remove all damaged porous materials with a twenty-four-inch margin to avoid mold growth.
- Improve airflow by opening doors and windows and moving furniture away from walls.
- When weather permits, open windows in your home to encourage outdoor airflow.
- Keep your basement well ventilated and make sure the sump pump works and there is no overflow or moisture soaking the carpets.
- Leave your bathroom fan on for thirty minutes after showering. Make sure the fan properly vents to the outside and vents are clear of debris and cleaned routinely.
- Dry your bathtub or shower with a squeegee after each use.
- Clean and repair damaged grout and apply a silicone or waterproof barrier to any exposed cracks in the tile around the shower or bathtub.

- Clean shower curtains, towels, rugs, and loofahs regularly. You can soak them in diluted bora.
- Use borax or other laundry additive for each load.

Sara swallowed the painful pill of mold remediation as only someone who had been fighting it her whole life could do. Her family took out a loan and initiated an extensive remediation to eradicate the source of mold in their home.

After remediation, as she tells it, "The nosebleeds and sleepwalking stopped, and my child stopped wetting the bed. We all felt so much better!"

Sara and her family's health is now much improved. She says, "I'm not perfect, or able to do everything I would like, but I see life through a new perspective and I am grateful."

A TERRIBLE SACRIFICE

Once I moved beyond my stubborn denial and implemented the Believe-Act-Wait recipe, it was like flipping a light switch. I called a certified inspector and met him at my office the very next day. We went to the basement of my office, and I watched in horror as he peeled off the baseboard and ran a scraper through the black mold that clung to the drywall underneath the trim. Knowing what I know now about how mold-sensitized my brain and body had become, I should have run out of the building right then, but instead I scraped a bit of mold myself, fascinated and terrified that my intuition was spot-on. Further inspection revealed not only that there was mold in the walls but that during the building's last remodel, the builders had cut some serious corners, including installation of soft bamboo flooring over the top of old musty carpet in the office where I saw patients every day. Ugh! Can you say mold sandwich?

In addition, my office sat directly over an unfinished crawl space; when the thousand-year flood washed through town, my clinic was a perfect nursery for a banner crop of Stachybotrys, one of the most toxic of molds.

I'd treated enough patients like Sara to know that there was no medicine or detox protocol that would heal me if I stayed in the moldy environment that made me sick. Once I got the results of the test confirming the mold was indeed the toxic Stachybotrys, I never again set foot in my beloved clinic. Not only did I walk away from my clinic, but I walked away from something that had been my constant companion for my entire life: my precious books.

Books had been my sanctuary from the farm environment even before I could read, and growing up, I thought I wanted to become a librarian. A book could transport me into other worlds and dimensions. Books fostered my love of learning, and they gave me a sense of security by helping me understand my environment. My floor-to-ceiling bookshelf was a centerpiece of my clinic, a diverse collection ranging from medical textbooks and journals to visionary and inspirational books written by the world's most revered illuminators of the soul's journey. My library was a physical representation of the happy coexistence of my spiritual and analytical self.

But the porous nature of paper makes it a perfect hideout for the airborne volatile organic compounds and mycotoxins that are emitted from a mold colony. When I walked away from my clinic that day, I was not only escaping an environment that was poisoning me but also walking away from what was, without a doubt, my single most precious material possession.

WHY NOW?

If the defiling mold reappears in the house after the stones have been torn out and the house scraped and plastered, [he] is to go and examine it and, if the mold has spread in the house, it is a persistent defiling mold; the house is unclean. It must be torn down—its stones, timbers and all the plaster—and taken out of the town to an unclean place.

LEVITICUS 14:43–44 (NIV), THREE THOUSAND YEARS AGO

So if mold has been around for thousands of years, why are we seeing more issues in buildings today? According to an article on mold and moisture in *Architect* magazine:

Building practices and materials have evolved at a rapid pace in the United States during the past century. Today the predominance of organic building materials, such as paper-faced drywall, wood framing, and plywood sheathing, provide a food source for mold growth. Also, increased energy costs and a limited supply of fuel have forced us to construct more energy-efficient buildings. Past construction practices allowed moisture from cooking, bathing, and other occupant activities to readily escape, along with conditioned air. According to the National Association of Home Builders (NAHB), we build homes that are 50% more energy efficient than 30 years ago. Sealing the building envelope against air loss is critical in achieving this performance. The problem arises when moisture and humidity levels are uncontrolled.[38]

In addition, toxic mold flourishes in the absence of competition, so in an old house rife with mold, it's likely that there are several distinct species of mold, which can keep the more dangerous varieties in check. That older construction is more porous and has various openings or cracks to the outside, allowing the home to breathe. In a modern home with a more robust seal between the interior and exterior environment, if toxic mold takes hold, without its primordial competitors or fresh outdoor airflow keeping it in check, the dangerous mold has free reign to grow uninhibited.

The mold spores can enter the house on building materials during construction, waiting in ambush for water intrusion from outside or even just a leaky washing machine. Modern homes are also commonly built with drywall rather than the brick, stone, and wood construction of yesteryear. Drywall makes for beautiful homes that are fast and inexpensive to build, but it's a mold nursery. Someone had the genius idea to add antifungals to indoor paints and drywall. Unfortunately, just as the unrestricted use of antibiotics in humans and livestock has resulted in antibiotic-resistant microbes, we are now seeing super-molds develop resistance to the antifungal materials, and indoor molds are showing a much greater aggressiveness and toxicity.

> The unintended consequences of antifungal and antibiotic use remind me of four insightful words my dad always says about farming: "Life flourishes despite us."

Need more guidance on mold treatment? You can download my free comprehensive mold guide at https://www.jillcarnahan.com/exposed-to-mold-now-what/

PLEASE DON'T TAKE MY BRAIN!

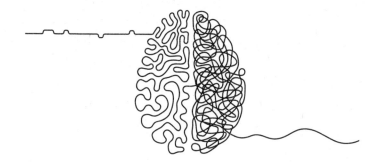

Mold sucks. After the original exposure, many patients become hypersensitized to subsequent exposures. Often called "unmasking," a patient may notice increased sensitivity during the detoxification process. Once they regain a bit of margin in their little toxin bucket, they may begin to notice chemicals and smells that never bothered them before. For a brief period of time, they may be hypersensitive to any subsequent mold exposure.

One day I was practicing kickboxing at a small hole-in-the-wall kind of gym that you find hidden between a Mexican restaurant and a nail salon. Had I been sparring, I would have gotten clobbered, but fortunately I was just doing a few roundhouse kicks to the bag. I didn't quite realize how off-kilter I was until I drove home. When I arrived home, I sideswiped my Lexus on the concrete pillar in the underground garage where I had parked every day for three years without incident, stripping the paint off the side of my shiny new vehicle.

Not long after, while driving home from a salon appointment after dark, I approached a police car that had pulled over another driver along the right-hand side of the interstate. Driving along, feeling disoriented (and a bit sleepy), I didn't perceive that the police car was not on the shoulder as I had thought but was partially in my lane. As I neared the flashing lights, I suddenly came to my senses and swerved to the left quickly, narrowly missing the terrified officer and her police car. I was shocked and startled but narrowly averted an accident. I was so discombobulated that moments later when the flashing lights appeared in my rearview mirror, my first thought was, "Oh, how thoughtful! She is making sure I am okay!" My smile turned to shock when she issued me a four-point ticket for careless driving. I really couldn't get too upset; it was my fault, but there was no way I was going to try to defend myself by explaining the real culprit— invisible mycotoxins in the salon I had just visited and the disorienting effect they had on my cognition.

Then there were the unexplained depressive symptoms I would have after attending a church on Sundays. I am naturally optimistic and happy, but for some odd reason after leaving this building, I felt like the entire world was crashing in, a dark feeling of hopelessness descending like a storm cloud over my psyche. I later found out that the building had a massive mold problem in the main lobby. I would often cry on the way home for no apparent reason and then fall into a deep sleep on the couch the moment I arrived home.

After a couple of these inexplicable events, I realized that the kick-boxing gym, the salon I had visited before the traffic violation, and the church I had attended all contained toxic mold. It's a scary thought, but I wonder: How many close calls and accidents on the road are caused by someone driving under the influence not of alcohol or drugs but mycotoxins? Or how many patients diagnosed with anxiety or depression are living in a home with mold that is worsening their symptoms?

Worse, when I was under the spell of that mycotoxin-induced mood alteration, I often lost my insight to understand that a toxin might be causing it. But thirty minutes after downing a few charcoal capsules and taking glutathione, both which aid detoxification, it was like the cloud lifted from my brain and the sun was shining again. I was always like, "Duh! It was the mold saboteur again!" Only afterward could I see clearly that the real culprit was exposure to mycotoxins.

One night after a mold hit, as tears flowed down my cheeks and soaked my hair and the pillow, I cried out, "God, you can take my ability to walk or my physical strength, but please, whatever you do, don't take my brain!" Toxic mold exposure not only took away my insight and understanding but also affected my focus and attention. I had never had symptoms of attention deficit disorder as a child (I could be lost in my own world for hours with laser focus), but under the influence of mycotoxins my brain would suddenly become like the talking dog, Dug, in the movie *Up* who said, "Squirrel!" and completely lost his mind. For the first few years after the flood, mold exposure would alter my ability to focus on completing a task, and it took me much longer to finish a project or write a blog article without interruptions. Having been through attacks on my breast with cancer and my colon with Crohn's, I was an experienced warrior and had the battle scars to prove it, but I knew that I would be lost without one of my most precious gifts: an analytical mind. I felt a sense of despair and wondered, *Will my laser focus ever fully return?*

There was a good reason for my fear. Mycotoxins, and even the nontoxic skeletal mold structure, can cause cognitive and emotional dysfunction.[39] Based on this, I now understand how mold hijacks the limbic system, the part of the brain responsible for recognizing a threat, and creates a subconscious chemical fear response. Instead of understanding that my feelings were being hijacked by a toxic insult that would soon pass, I felt as if I were on a plane that had lost all air pressure and had started dropping from the sky: pure fear, no logic, pure limbic response.

In animal studies, lesions in the limbic region are associated with irrational fears, feelings of strangeness or unreality, wishing to be alone, and sadness. A feeling of being out of touch with or out of control of one's feelings and thoughts, not unlike that described by my patients with chemical sensitivity and mold exposure, may be perceived. Some report feeling "spacey" or that "the camera isn't on" unless they make an enormous effort to focus their attention. The vague term *brain fog* is often what patients tell me they experience after mold exposure. We also know from research that the olfactory system (breathing in through the nose, which is one of the main routes mycotoxins enter our body) is linked directly to the hypothalamus, which governs the limbic system. The olfactory system, hypothalamus, and limbic system pathways explain the neural circuitry by which adverse food, chemical, and mold reactions could trigger certain neural, psychological, and psychiatric abnormalities.[40]

Even though I understood that this was just another "mold hit," my frontal cortex didn't get the message and responded as if it were a new life-threatening event, changing me temporarily and making me behave almost like a different person. This is no surprise.

> When mold hijacks our limbic system
> and bypasses our more rational
> frontal cortex, we may behave in ways
> that seem completely irrational.

And worse, when mold is messing with our minds it is hard for us to perceive in ways that are easily understood or communicated to others in verbal language.

I realized that in order to help my patients truly heal from mold toxicity, this PTSD-like limbic response must be addressed just as carefully as the physical symptoms that mold causes. I frequently prescribe many ways of addressing limbic dysfunction to my patients (see sidebar) at their first visit. Addressing this very real chemical trauma is critical in the healing process, and no matter how well adjusted you are, it may be one of the most important steps in healing.

Limbic Retraining Suggestions

Recommended Reading
- *Accessing the Healing Power of the Vagus Nerve* by Stanley Rosenberg
- *The Brain That Changes Itself* by Norman Doidge
- *Breaking the Habit of Being Yourself* by Joe Dispenza
- *What Happened to You?* by Oprah Winfrey and Bruce Perry
- *The Body Keeps the Score* by Bessel A. van der Kolk
- *Scattered Minds* by Gabor Maté
- *Transforming Trauma* by James Gordon

Guided Programs and Practices
- *BrainTap* app
- *Safe and Sound Protocol* by Stephen Porges
- *Dynamic Neural Retraining System* by Annie Hopper
- Gupta Program *Brain Retraining*
- *HeartMath Program*

Restorative Therapies
- Neurofeedback
- Medical hypnosis
- Neurolinguistic programming
- Cranial sacral therapy
- Integrative Manual Therapy (IMT)
- Somatic experiencing therapy
- Emotional Freedom Technique or "tapping"
- Frequency specific microcurrent
- Breath work like Buteyko breathing

- Listen to binaural beats to calm the nervous system
- Practice flow (see sidebar "Ten Ways To Experience More Flow" on page 140)

INVISIBLE EVIL

Stachybotrys, the same strain of mold I had in my office, has a reputation for casting a sinister darkness over the sufferer. One of my mold patients learned that the house where she'd been exposed to Stachybotrys had been the site of two homicides and one suicide, totally unrelated to each other. After watching the horrible impacts of mold on her family's health, she contacted me and begged me to treat her daughter, who was suffering the severe effects of mold-related illness. Now she is convinced of two things: one, I saved her daughter's life, and two, those grizzly deaths of the former tenants in her mold-infested home had something to do with the malicious mycotoxins that lurked inside.

Could it be?

My speculations on the "personalities" of different molds are based on anecdotal evidence, but mold is a fungus, and fungi have been instrumental in the development of numerous powerful pharmaceuticals, including penicillin, strong immunosuppressive drugs, and the widely used cholesterol-lowering statins. For thousands of years people have known of the hallucinogenic qualities of several kinds of fungi, using them as recreational drugs as well as a gateway to enlightenment and spiritual experience. Is it possible that some of the mold growing in buildings releases chemicals that can cause altered states specific to the mold species and the types of mycotoxins they produce? Of this I have no doubt.

When I was exposed to mycotoxins from mold, I experienced a specific set of symptoms based on the type of mold exposure.

Chaetomium, one of the most toxic molds, produces toxic metabolites called chaetoglobosins. Exposure to this mold made me irresistibly sleepy and completely stole my motivation. I'd sometimes have to pull over while driving and take a nap—not a refreshing Saturday afternoon kind of nap but more like Sleeping Beauty after she pricked her finger on the evil stepmother's spindle. I would be stone-cold out. I nicknamed it the "narcoleptic mold" based on my experience. Later I learned that the Chaetomium toxins caused a sudden drop in my blood pressure (which often registered as low as 80/50) due to a genetic variation in a gene called iNOS and caused a form of postural orthostatic tachycardia in which my blood pressure would drop so low it was impossible to remain upright—or awake! Some of my friends even joked about having me visit their home to see if they had a mold issue, as if I were some kind of mold dog. While I have no interest in changing professions, the truth is, due to my extreme sensitivities, I am a very accurate human mold detector.

Scouring medical journals for articles on mold illness, I have come across some fascinating (and horrifying) reports of mycotoxin-induced psychosis, including "delusional parasitosis or infestation," which is essentially a hallucination of infestation with parasites or inanimate objects (yeah, like bugs-crawling-under-the-skin kind of horrible). Several researchers have looked into the possibility that ergot poisoning, a condition associated with seizures and psychosis and caused by a mold found in rye, was behind the bewitched behavior that led to the Salem witch trials and murders. In the 1700s, just fifty years later, the fits of madness associated with ergot poisoning were thought to be a mark of holy, not demonic, possession. We've come a long way in understanding human health since then, but we still have much to learn about the many toxic metabolites produced by mold species.

Steps to Heal from Mold-Related Illness

At first it can be totally overwhelming to learn that mold may be contributing to your symptoms, but I have had success with thousands of patients in reversing the mold-related symptoms with these simple steps.

- Avoid mold exposure and remove yourself from the environment if mold is present.
- Get further testing to determine the extent of exposure and what else may be contributing to your symptoms. Rule out other causes (see sidebar "What to Do If You Suspect Mold-Related Illness" on page 165).
- Purchase a high-quality air filter for your bedroom and home.
- Follow a low mold/low-histamine diet
  - Avoid foods that commonly contain mycotoxins. Some of these include corn, barley, wheat, peanuts, rye, cottonseed, chilies, spices, dried fruit, cocoa, coffee, bread, black pepper, and alcoholic beverages.
  - Avoid sugar in all forms, processed foods, gluten, and grains, which are often contaminated with mycotoxins.
  - Enjoy mold-free coffee like Purity coffee; organic pasture-raised meat; low-carb vegetables, nuts, and seeds (use caution with peanuts, cashews, and pistachios); and healthy fats, like coconut, avocado, and extra virgin olive oil.

- Support your liver and gallbladder with detox supplements like liposomal glutathione, N-acetylcysteine, alpha-lipoic acid, milk thistle, Calcium D-glucorate, glycine, glutamine, taurine, sulphorophanes, ascorbic acid, and bitters.
- Use detox binders like activated charcoal, bentonite clay, chitosan, chlorella, glucomannan, humic and fulvic acids, modified citrus pectin, prebiotics and probiotics, Saccharomyces boulardii, and zeolite.
- Adopt other practices to enhance and support your detox pathways.
  - Drink alkaline or mineral water with electrolytes to hydrate your system.
  - Use an infrared sauna regularly.
  - Use IV glutathione and nicotinamide adenine dinucleotide (NAD+).
  - Use dry brushing to support lymphatics.
  - Take Epsom salt baths.
  - Use coffee enemas or castor oil packs.
  - Rinse sinuses with a saline neti pot or use a diluted solution of colloidal silver or grapefruit seed extract if fungal/mold colonization is present.

For more information on my favorite supplements to treat mold, visit www.ReadUnexpected.com/Resources.

UNCONSCIOUS UNCOUPLING

Looking back, I can see so clearly how mold illness impacted my insight, my coping skills, and my emotional capacity to tend to the needs of the loved ones in my life. In the year following my mold exposure, I was in complete survival mode. I was terrified that I would lose everything I had worked so hard to build, and so I poured what little energy I had into keeping my clinic going, moving my entire office and staff to a clean temporary space, and finding a more permanent location. I stopped going out with friends or doing anything but the barest necessities of life. I was so traumatized and emotionally overwhelmed that I was not consciously aware of the massive strain on my marriage. And clearly, I had no idea how to ask for help or support, so I continued suffering silently. Had I known what was coming, I might have paid more attention.

> Anything that causes a prolonged inflammatory reaction in the body can affect a person's decision-making in dramatic ways.

As I described earlier, the limbic effects of mold on our feelings and behavior include irrational fears, detachment, depersonalization, wishing to be alone, and often a sense of overwhelm or hopelessness. This leads to an unconscious and very subtle detachment from reality, which is probably an adaptive coping mechanism for this awful illness. Rapidly growing evidence indicates that chemical toxins like mold and mycotoxins may affect mood and behavior for years if there is no intervention.

Under the influence of a significant trauma (both psychological and chemical) like mold exposure, we lose our ability to articulate what is happening to us, our thoughts become scattered, and our memories of the event become confused and disjointed. When another subsequent traumatic experience triggers these memories and scattered thoughts, we revert to the emotional patterns that we developed during the original trauma, reacting to the present based on our experienced trauma of the past. In this way, unresolved trauma builds on itself, like a wagon wheel creating a deep track in the soft earth, reinforcing its effect on the psyche with every new stressor, and we can suffer emotional pain from events long past without ever understanding why. If you have ever had a day of unexpected sadness and then later realized it was the anniversary of a tragic event or death of someone you loved, you know what I mean. As physician and *New York Times* bestselling author Bessel A. van der Kolk says, "The body keeps score…" and it often remembers sadness and trauma that we have consciously forgotten over the years.

Aaron made a movie about love. I was practicing medicine in a clinic with a mission of love. We loved one another deeply and believed in the strength of our relationship. But deep inside we were being devoured by lack of emotional vulnerability and support, just when we needed it most. We didn't know how to ask for what we needed most of all during this time: connection, understanding, and unconditional love.

Embrace GRACE

We all need reminders on how to continue showing up as our fully authentic selves and practicing loving-kindness. That is why I created this acronym to remind me to practice GRACE every day. You can use this as a reminder to show up with compassion and understanding for yourself and others.

Gentleness: In a world on edge, choose to show up with kindness and gentleness. This holds immense power for healing our fellow humans and our world.

Resilience: Resilience is the ability to recover or bounce back. Make it a habit of asking yourself, Will this matter in five minutes or five hours or five days? Ask yourself what really matters, then align yourself with the things that do. Believe in your ability to figure it out and overcome any obstacle.

Acceptance: Let go of judgment and learn to welcome others just where they are with unconditional love and acceptance. Most important, learn to accept yourself exactly as you are, flaws and all.

Compassion: Seek first to understand others and remember that everyone is on their own journey at their own pace of healing, and each deserves loving-kindness and compassion. Practice assuming the best about your partner, family members, and coworkers.

Empowerment: Show up with true authenticity without apologizing for who you are or making yourself smaller. Let go of concerns over what others will think and instead live your life with vibrancy and joy!

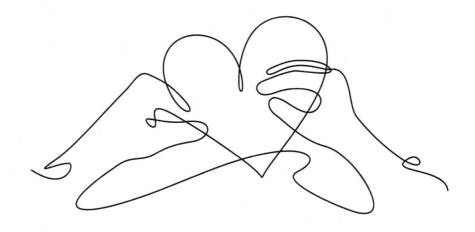

CHAPTER 7

Choosing Unconditional Love

There is no greater power in Heaven or on Earth than pure, unconditional love. The nature of the God force, the unseen intelligence in all things, which causes the material world and is the center of both the spiritual and physical plane, is best described as pure, unconditional love.

—WAYNE DYER

KISSING BOYS

Do you remember your first kiss?

We all have a clumsy start with love, and mine was no different. It was a long journey from my first awkward kiss in the fifth grade to understanding the power of unconditional love as the most potent tool for true healing. It all began on a Sunday in May near the end of my fifth grade school year. The fifth through eighth grades had gathered for a Sunday school picnic in the park, complete with burgers and soda and games at the community pool. There was a large horse trough filled with soda on ice. We dipped our hands into the ice water to grab our favorite soda and shiver with the painfully cold sensation as we tried to fish out our favorite flavor as quickly as possible.

I had a crush on one of my classmates named Mark, and after passing notes to each other through schoolmates so we could avoid the terrible embarrassment of actually talking to each other, we were finally "going together." We didn't go anywhere together, and I had yet to even hold his hand, but that was what we called the puppy love crush in junior high school. I had certainly been feeling pressure from my girlfriends to kiss the boy. That afternoon, sitting next to each other under the large oak tree outside the park building, swinging our legs in unison, he made his move.

He leaned over, placed his hand on top of mine, and planted a moist kiss on my lips, not unlike those I would get from my little brother. My first kiss was a bit of a disappointment, but I felt relieved that it was over. I had done it and lived to tell my girlfriends, of course, exaggerating the details just a little in the story.

At thirteen I had my second taste of romantic love during an encounter at a hotel in St. Louis during a school event. After the event, several of my friends and I were invited to hang out with some of the kids from other schools. As I walked in the room, I was drawn to a sixteen-year-old boy with a chiseled face, blond spiked hair, and sparkling blue eyes that locked on mine from across the room. He was a foreign exchange student named Hans who had a delicious German accent. I giggled as he mispronounced English words in a way I found quite appealing. Later I fell in the parking lot as we were running to the pool, cutting my palm so deeply that I should have had stitches, but I wasn't about to be deterred from my evening with Hans. As the evening wore on, we swam in the pool and then moved on to the hot tub, where he planted a kiss squarely on my lips. This time my insides melted with new sensations, and I wanted more. He obviously did too, and we sat and talked and kissed between words. I felt his tongue in my mouth, and I realized to my delight I would now be able to tell my girlfriends that I was the first one of us to be French kissed!

As we stepped out of the hot tub, he took my hand and suggested we go for a walk. We dried off, and he guided me the back way up a quiet staircase. He gently pushed me up against the wall and started kissing me much more intensely, and I began to feel just a little bit afraid. He closed his eyes and groaned slightly. Although I didn't want to stop, my hand was still bleeding from the nasty fall, and the throbbing wound reminded me that good girls do not make out in dark staircases. I gently pushed him away and left to go back to my room alone. Looking down at my right palm today, I can still see the deep one-inch scar and am reminded of the French kiss with a German boy named Hans. But that wasn't love either.

In high school I went out a couple of times with a guy named Jim, a simple farm boy from the town next to mine. He didn't say much. He was terribly shy but sweet with dirty blond hair, green eyes, and a southern drawl. We would sit in his bedroom, chastely watching James Bond movies. I think he was afraid to hold my hand at first, but finally glancing my way, he reached over, blushing slightly, and put his sweaty palm in mine. I was attracted to his kindness and vulnerability. He told me he loved me on our second or third date and I got nervous, and that was the end of it. Then there was Alex, tall and lanky, with bright blue eyes, blue jeans, a pickup truck, and cowboy boots. I know it sounds like a terrible country-western song, but I crashed my parents' van and then lost my virginity to him.

I was driving home late one afternoon from an appointment, feeling a bit sleepy. An icy rain was falling. I stopped at the stop sign in front of the only highway in the small town of Roanoke but neglected to look both directions properly and proceeded into the intersection. Seconds later, a fully loaded semitruck going 65 mph hit me just behind my driver's door. My parents' conversion van spun around twice, careened into the parking lot across the road, and totaled a pickup truck before crashing through the front window of the local pizza parlor. The last thing I remember is seeing the headlights of the semitruck coming directly at me. When I regained consciousness, an oxygen mask was being placed over my face in the ambulance. All I know is that angels were watching out for me that afternoon because I escaped with only a minor concussion.

The very next evening, still groggy from the concussion, I had a date with Alex, and while we were kissing passionately, he pulled out a condom and it was over. Yes, just like that, I lost what I had considered a very precious part of me. I was so ashamed. I had really had no intention of going that far and had always anticipated that I would save myself for my wedding night. Years later, my friend gasped as I shared this story with her and said, "Oh, Jill, you were likely still quite traumatized from the concussion and in no condition to make that decision." Looking back, I feel sadness for that tough but sensitive girl who was just looking for affirmation that she was lovable. I broke up with Alex shortly thereafter. We'd gone all the way, but not all the way to love, and certainly nowhere near unconditional love.

SHOCKWAVES

I'll never forget that day late in May, just days before my fortieth birthday, when my carefully crafted house of cards came crashing down. I flew out to meet my husband for his father's funeral. He greeted me with a cold harshness and contempt that I had never felt from him before. I chalked it all up to the monumental stress and grief he must have been under as he was getting ready to bury his father after an unexpected death. The first taste of fear tickled my lips when he picked me up at the airport. I tripped getting into the car. Instead of helping me, he glowered and yelled, "Hurry up!" Normally, we would greet each other with a warm embrace, but this time all I felt was his anger and frustration. Even his normally sparkling blue eyes were dark and wouldn't meet my own.

After the funeral, I left to speak at a conference, and we reunited at home a week later. He opened the door, and as I ran to welcome him home, I immediately detected something was dramatically wrong. I stopped short, as if there were a physical barrier between us, and my heart lurched in fear. Instead of the warm, loving man whom I had known for nearly twenty years, I was staring into blank, expressionless eyes, and a hollow voice I'd never heard before said, "Jill, I don't love you anymore."

> **The brutal feeling of his rejection was the beginning of my own awakening.**

I had previously been so good at believing my own Pollyanna version of reality that I had never really examined my dysfunctional coping mechanisms or flawed beliefs. Instead, I had carefully crafted a version of reality that hid the cracks and signs of disconnect, ignoring anything that was uncomfortable or didn't fit into the delicately crafted version of the perfect marriage I had conjured up in my mind. Like one last teetering China teacup that's added to the carefully balanced stack and causes the entire tower to come crashing down, that one day changed my life and my version of reality forever. And the truth was, until that moment, I had believed every bit of it. In order to cope with the devastating divorce I never once saw coming, I had to dig deeper than I'd ever gone, into my family of origin and my beliefs about myself and about others and the world. Instead of blaming Aaron for everything, I knew I needed to discover what parts of my own behaviors and beliefs had led to this shocking situation.

I sought solace in the things that had always comforted me—having coffee with girlfriends, going on long hikes in the mountains, and spending time in prayer and meditation, but every time I came back to reality, the same questions plagued me: How had this happened? Who was I as an individual after twenty years of being in a partnership? Could I survive alone? Was I still lovable? Was there something wrong with me? I had devoted my heart and life to one man and never once thought about divorce as an option. I'd overcome so many other challenges, but nothing had prepared me for this pain of heart and soul that rocked me to the core.

> I was an expert at solving medical
> mysteries of environmental toxicity,
> but I had neglected to look at my own
> emotional and relational toxicity.

But even in the darkest times, I knew there was reason to look for the light. In the words of Yung Pueblo, "Heartbreak is not always a sad ending; sometimes it sets in motion a profound transformation. It can open the door to absolutely loving yourself, becoming more emotionally mature and learning what type of partner would actually support your happiness." Intuitively I knew, from my own experiences and from watching my patients overcome the most dire situations, that challenges held the greatest opportunity for growth. The question was, how in the world could I work through the fear, doubt, discouragement, and complete and utter abandonment that I was currently feeling?

Sometimes we can't fix what has been broken.
The act of surrender is accepting that truth.
—*MIGUEL RUIZ JR., A MEXICAN AUTHOR*
OF TOLTEC SPIRITUALIST TEXTS

LOVE NEURONS

In the painful months following the divorce, I found myself in a relationship with a retired police officer who turned out to be an abusive stalker with borderline personality and bipolar disorder. He moved into the apartment complex next to mine, which was convenient until one day he slammed me against a wall in anger. I was finally beginning to value myself and learn how to set boundaries, and so after consulting with a therapist who helped me understand this was abusive behavior, I filed a restraining order at the local courthouse. While driving by on my way home a few days later, my heart nearly stopped as I saw the flashing lights of an ambulance and two cop cars in front of his apartment. I gasped with shock, but my intuition knew what had happened before they told me. The police found him dead in his apartment with an empty bottle of opioids on his nightstand. Despite the abuse, my heart was torn with sadness because I felt that no human being, no matter what they have done, should endure the type of suffering that makes them want to end their life.

A few months later, I dated a man who was a convicted felon and alcoholic who fit eighteen of twenty clinical criteria of psychopathy. Clearly, I knew none of this when we started dating. I know that sounds like a horrific want ad ("SWF seeks psychopathic alcoholic felon"), but I simply had no idea what I was getting into or how my past experiences and empathetic heart made me so vulnerable to the seduction of the wrong type of man. I still had so much to learn.

All this, just when I thought I was waking up.

Previously, I was so adept at seeing only the good side of things that I didn't know I needed to wake up. After the divorce, I realized that perhaps my sanguine view of life was a bit skewed. I was ready to go deeper than I'd ever gone and look harder than I had ever looked at myself and my foundational beliefs. I was no stranger to personal growth and transformation, but I was at a point in life where I needed to first shred my current version of reality and reexamine my long-held beliefs to see if they would really hold up in the second half of my life. I had overcome multiple life-threatening illnesses and become an expert in functional medicine and was a sought-after educator at medical conferences around the world. I received feedback every day from my patients, thanking me for changing their lives, but I was still a bit of a mess on the personal level, and I didn't even feel like a hot one.

We've long understood that our intimate relationships are powerful mediators of our emotions, but we've only just begun to realize how much they influence our physical health. Those who have recently been separated from loved ones account for one-third more acute illnesses and physician visits than married people. Furthermore, marital divorce or separation is the single most significant sociodemographic predictor of stress-related physical illness. The influence is also measurable; the same study found that women separated within the previous year had worse immune function than sociodemographically matched married women.[41] Neuroscientists have called the neural network that is stimulated by loss of love the "panic circuit." It is closely related to the pain circuit but also includes grief and sorrow.[42] The mediator for this system is the opioid system, the oxytocin-based response that eventually can make us feel good again through the haze of pain. It's why opioids are so addictive and work so well to soothe pain. The commonalities between opioid addiction and social dependence are stunning. As Jaak Panksepp wrote in his authoritative book, *Affective Neuroscience,*

To be alone and lonely, to be without nurturance or a consistent source of gratification, are among the worst and most commonplace emotional pains humans must endure. . . . Love is in part, the neurochemically based positive feeling that negates those negative feelings.[43]

Essentially, Panksepp is saying that unconditional love is the antidote to pain and suffering. Love is how we get through the inevitable pains of life and climb out of that pit of despair that every one of us has looked into, a dark hole that can be tricky to climb out of. It's no wonder I sought out some semblance of love and affection (albeit a very false version) from the wrong types of men, one who was physically abusive and the other emotionally manipulative.

While I was certainly confused in my perception of love, I had experienced unconditional love in my life and was no stranger to its healing power. My ex-husband had given his all to support me through cancer and Crohn's, risking his job, shaving his head, and baring his soul in front of Dr. Kuske to get me into the "Shish Kaboob" therapy. It made no difference to him that I may never look the same or even survive cancer. That was truly unconditional love or, as the Greeks called it, *agape*, the kind of love that holds the highest regard for another person.

Humanist psychologist Carl Rogers coined a similar term, *unconditional positive regard* toward another. He said that all individuals needed an environment that provided them with the qualities of genuineness, authenticity, openness, self-disclosure, acceptance, empathy, and approval, or unconditional love.[44]

Some of the most profound lessons I learned about love were in the throes of the difficulties I encountered in my post-divorce relationships. I am sure you are wondering, *What were you thinking, Jill?!* Well, in my defense, I had just come out of a twenty-year marriage with all the dating experience of a nineteen-year-old. I was codependent and completely naive and trusting, an empathetic target for narcissists with what proved to be the fatal flaw of seeing only the good and ignoring the danger that existed in each of these relationships.

I frequently hear from professional women and men like myself who are successful in the business world but have had difficulty with romantic relationships because of a lack of boundaries, feelings of unworthiness, and lack of love and respect for themselves. In time I realized I could only allow myself to be treated in the context of what I believed about myself on the most basic level. If I didn't believe I was worthy of loving-kindness, I would allow terrible mistreatment because it fit into what I believed I was deserving of.

> Until we choose self-love and compassion,
> we will continue to allow ourselves to
> enter into toxic, unhealthy relation-
> ships because we don't believe we
> are worthy of love and respect.

These are very painful lessons to learn, but once I understood my value as a woman worthy of the greatest love and respect, I could never again let others mistreat me. There was transforming power in learning to love and value myself first. I practiced by adopting new habits I had never thought to do before, like dressing up and taking myself out to a fancy dinner or museum or buying myself a weekly bouquet of a dozen fresh roses. This experience helped me craft my own definition of unconditional love:

Freely and generously offering loving-kindness to everyone and everything, without any limits or conditions attached. It begins by showing the same unconditional loving-kindness and compassion to ourselves and by accepting all the parts of ourselves, even those we may have previously deemed unworthy, because without this, we cannot experience true healing.

Don't despair if you recognize you are in an unhealthy relationship. You have the power to choose again every day. I'll never forget what my friend Cheryl Gray once told me, "You know, Jill, you walk along a street and one day you fall into a pothole. The next day you walk along the same street and fall in again. And this goes on repeatedly, over and over until finally you decide to take a different street. But until you are ready, you will go the same way and fall into the same hole over and over again. But one day . . . one day you will take a new route and you will never again walk on that street or fall in the same hole." Yes, it is true. Sadly, sometimes it takes falling more than once, but once we finally change, we can never again go back.

DADDY'S GIRL

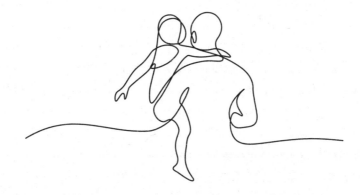

Trauma doesn't always have a capital T. No matter the severity, in order to survive emotionally, we often repaint a beautiful picture of our past in order to protect the ones who may have harmed us. In doing so, we betray our own selves. Have you ever felt as if there were no room for your desires, your needs, or your passions? Have you ever felt like you didn't belong? Did you ever feel unsafe and unprotected as a child? Did you put on an armor of strength and bravery, vowing to take care of yourself so that you had to rely on no one, lest you be betrayed? I know this little girl. She is me.

Because she adopted hypervigilance early in life, it is difficult for her to let down her guard and rest. She finds herself unable to receive any loving care or nurturing that comes her way. She feels she must always "perform," for she believes that it is only by constantly achieving that she is worthy of receiving love.

But at the core, all she really desires is love. And beneath this shell of bravery is the shame she feels when her humanity sneaks through the cracks of the mask she so carefully crafted to show the world she is strong and capable. Yet she must risk becoming vulnerable in order to heal or surrender to the sheer exhaustion that will eventually come from lack of rest. It is only when she is alone that she can give herself what she needs—but only when no one is watching. Receiving loving care from others is the most difficult thing to accept, but it is also the only thing that will heal her lonely heart. She wants to be seen and known and held in love, but she doesn't believe she is allowed to have needs or desires, and so this great internal conflict ensues.

As you can see, resting and receiving exposes the vulnerability that I spent a lifetime suppressing. But after a life of working this hard, resting only when I was knocked down by illness, and framing my entire perspective of my worthiness of love around achievement, I intuitively knew that if I didn't try to understand the core wounds around this illusion, I would reap the rewards of sheer exhaustion and burnout.

I started the healing process with something I knew would be well received. I wrote a letter to the man I admire most in the world, who I knew would understand and appreciate my efforts at healing, who had been a solid anchor and inspiration in my life since the day I was born, who had shown me how to give my best every single day: my daddy. I sat down in my favorite coffee shop and poured out my heart, typing a letter to him on the computer. As I typed, tears fell and soaked my keyboard. I told him how much he meant to me, how he had shaped and influenced my life in a million positive ways over the years. I asked him to help me heal the sensitive and vulnerable seven-year-old little girl deep inside who needed to be reminded that her daddy loved her and thought she was special even when she couldn't work as hard as her brothers. I said some things I had wanted to say for my entire life but never felt comfortable expressing. I went to the most vulnerable place I have ever gone, knowing my dad would have the love and compassion to help me heal old wounds. After I wrote the letter, I took a deep breath and with a little anxiety at feeling so vulnerable, I hit the send button. It didn't take long to get a response. He texted me shortly after and said, "Jill, I got your email and appreciate your letter so much. If you could, would you give me twenty-four hours to respond properly?" I was shaking and typed, "Yes, Daddy."

It didn't take long. The next afternoon when I saw my father's name in my inbox, I couldn't even open the email. I began sobbing and shaking and fell to the floor, knowing what I was about to read would forever change me. True to my expectation, my father wrote some of the most precious words I had ever read, what I had longed to hear as a seven-year-old. He went on to explain that unbeknownst to me, the year I turned seven he almost lost the farm and spent many long, sleepless nights worried and praying that he wouldn't lose all he owned and plunge the family into dire straits. My sensitive seven-year-old empath soul felt his distress and grief, and somehow I had thought it was my fault that my daddy was upset. He shared his own struggles with profound vulnerability in response to my own and ended with saying how much he loved me back then and still did today, how he was proud of me and thought I was the most wonderful daughter a father could have. I know it may seem like a small thing, but prior to writing him that letter, I realized that some of my poor choices in men stemmed from a wounded little girl who was longing to be reminded how much her daddy loved her and thought she was precious, special, and unique. My father and I have always had a loving relationship, and there was no strain between us. But this deeply precious, vulnerable exchange, for me in my forties and for him in his seventies, forever changed my relationship with my father in an amazing way, and it forever changed how I would date and what kind of men I would choose from that moment on.

I often wonder how many broken little girls or boys are walking around in forty- or fifty-year-old bodies making poor choices in relationships based on fractured parts of themselves. How many people could find profound healing by the simple act of writing a letter to their daddy? If this is speaking to you, dear reader, I hope you put this book down immediately and go do what needs to be done in order to heal your little girl (or boy) wounds. I promise you, it could change your life.

MY GRANDMOTHER'S GIFT

Several weeks later, I set up a Zoom date with my dear Grandma Farney, in part to reach out from the isolation of the pandemic but also to dig even deeper into the mysteries of my health and relationship challenges in light of my ancestors and their history. The computer screen flickered with a face I know and love so well, still young eyes smiling, surrounded by the wrinkled map of her long life etched into her face. I apologized to my grandma for not being able to be there in person, and she replied, "No, this is wonderful! All this modern stuff; I can't even absorb it all."

It's hard to fathom the changes she's seen in her life, from growing up canning chickens before freezers were invented to using a computer the size of a magazine to see and speak with her granddaughter in real time a thousand miles away. No wonder she was as thrilled to see me on a laptop screen as she would have been in person. She returned the favor and then some—my grandma proceeded to tell me the story of a toxicity that blew my mind, winding its way from a decision of my great-grandparents all the way down to me.

Like me, my grandmother spent her childhood on a farm in what would seem to be one of the healthiest environments on earth. She worked hard every day as, in her words, her dad's "right-hand man." Also like me, she was blessed with a muscular frame and felt the need to hide it. She wore overalls, work boots, and a flannel shirt. She would braid her long, thick hair and wrap the braids around the top of her head and tuck them under a hat. It worked; more than one of the neighbors, after seeing her working in the field, thought there was a new man hired to work on the farm.

These were the years of the Dust Bowl and the Great Depression. Working hard every day but having enough to eat was a luxury reserved for the lucky ones. "At times we pretty much ate only chicken, eggs, and potatoes," she said. "If we had a dime to go buy a loaf of bread, that was really something, but we always had enough to eat."

When she was a teenager, her dad decided to leave the farm and start a car dealership in town. He made more money, but the cost was the health of generations. They built an apartment upstairs from the garage, which was both a showroom and a repair shop—a toxic environment including lead and benzene in the gasoline and diesel and asbestos dust from the car brake assemblies. The volatile fumes almost certainly contributed to the lung cancer and liver cirrhosis that killed my great-grandparents (neither of whom smoke or drank) and were the likely culprit behind my grandma's worst memory: giving her little sister a final large morphine dose to end her suffering from metastatic melanoma at the early age of forty.

How does a person get over something as horrific as this? If my grandmother's tears while telling me the story forty years later are any indication, you don't really ever get over it. But if her genuine laughter and happiness in the rest of our conversation are any indication, the overriding emotion of her life is joy, not sadness.

At the time my grandmother told me about the toxic garage, she was nearly ninety years old and as healthy and full of life as she was as a little girl. She didn't succumb to the illnesses that ravaged her family. Perhaps it is because she was old enough to leave the apartment to work every day, so her toxic load wasn't as great as the rest of her family. Or perhaps someone needed to tell my family's story so I could pass it on. I'll never know why. But I believe there is meaning in her story. And mine. And yours. And knowing there is always meaning and purpose to be found makes a difference.

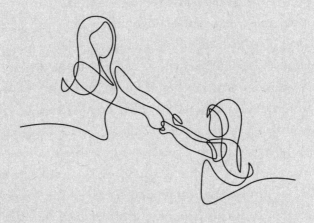

The Benefits of Trauma

Clearly, trauma is difficult and can have lasting effects on our mind and body. I would never wish trauma on anyone. However, here are some of the ways that trauma turns into a powerful, transformative force in our lives.

1. Creates resilience
2. Teaches humor/taking life less seriously
3. Encourages empathy
4. Increases wisdom and understanding
5. Improves problem-solving skills and creativity
6. Allows for introspection and growth

My grandmother was exposed to a heavy amount of toxicity as a child, which was almost certainly passed on to my mother and to me in some form. We spoke of joy, trauma, love, fear, and faith. We shared laughter and tears, and the point of every conversation was the same: healing. One of the most important things we learn from those in the last decades of life is the importance of making peace with others and freely giving love and forgiveness while we each still draw breath.

> Perhaps the most important question we each can ask ourselves before we turn the page is, Is there someone in my life I need to forgive?

FENTANYL LOLLIPOPS

Around the same time my marriage was dying, I met a couple who demonstrated one of the most powerful healing experiences of unconditional love I have ever witnessed.

It started with a call from Alyssa, who was curious to know if I might be able to help her husband, Burke, who had been suffering from inexplicable and almost unendurable difficulties since he was a teenager. I knew I would be facing a challenging case, but I had no idea that their love story would take them around the world and result in unexpected healing that makes even my own seem simple by comparison.

Seventeen years earlier, Burke had been winning every ski race he entered in one of the most challenging and prestigious ski programs in Colorado. He was preparing for the national championship competition over spring break when he woke up one morning to incredible pain from sores the size of quarters lining his mouth and throat. The doctors said it was infectious mononucleosis or "mono" and that it would go away.

"My life exploded," Burke recalled. "I went from being a ski-racing champion, having never smoked pot or drank, to being handed Percocet so I could go to school for the day."

The pain was so severe that attending school became impossible, and he was taken to the Children's Hospital in Denver. His dad had to carry him through the door of the hospital. Since he couldn't swallow, nutrients delivered via IV kept him alive. Eventually he was able to return to school, but the doctors said he would need to continue to use the IV if he couldn't eat.

"I was sixteen years old," Burke said. "There was no way I was going to be at school eating my lunch through a tube."

With teenage pride and a natural gift of tenacity, he forced himself to eat through extreme pain. By the time Burke was a junior in high school, the sores in his mouth had eaten away his tonsils and uvula and he was consuming dangerously high doses of opiates just to get through each day. One day he'd had enough and decided to wean himself off the pain medication. Burke stopped using the fentanyl lollipops that had been compounded so that the pain medication could reach his oral mucosa, which was completely ulcerated and raw. While his friends skied and discovered the freedom of driver's licenses, he learned of the tortures of opiate withdrawal. But he soldiered on, attending college at the University of Colorado in Boulder. By then he had become an expert at hiding pain and presenting himself to the world as if he had no problems.

"I just wanted to be a kid," he said. "But there is nothing like going on a date and sneaking away to spray your mouth with benzocaine just so you can talk."

After graduating with a degree in psychology, he met Alyssa. She fell in love with the troubled young man even though he'd been told he would never have kids due to the damage from the disease. But it wasn't until after they moved in together that she learned the extent of the suffering he'd been hiding from everyone, including his own parents. Alyssa fueled by love and the firm belief that there had to be a solution to Burke's troubles, devoted her life to helping him heal. She became his advocate, insisting his medical team take his complaints seriously and help him find answers. It was her persistence that finally led her to call my office.

By the time she called me, I had been working for fifteen years as what my colleagues often refer to jokingly as a "resort doctor," or the doctor of last resort. After doing my homework, my intuition knew the likely culprit: tick-borne infections, like Borrelia burgdorferi, and coinfections.

Burke wasn't convinced. He'd already tested negative for Lyme disease through the standard western blot test. In addition, seventeen years of having doctors get it wrong had left him with little faith. For Alyssa, however, my suggestion was a glimmer of hope for the man she loved. They went back to their mountain home, and during a slow day at work, Alyssa compiled and printed out five pages of common Lyme disease symptoms resulting not only from the infection but the inflammatory cytokines produced by a weakened immune state. She and Burke sat on the sofa that night and went through the list. He fit over ninety percent of them.

"After reading the list, I was in full-blown tears," Burke said. "For the first time, somebody not only sort of got it but hit the nail on the head. For the first time in my life, I had a glimpse of hope." I hear this echo so many times when patients, feeling desperate and ignored by the medical system for years, find hope when they are finally given a framework for their illness. Pain isn't just from illness; it includes not knowing why you are suffering, being shuffled from doctor to doctor, and being told you are crazy or need an antidepressant.

I suggested more advanced, sensitive, and slightly more expensive testing, including Immunoblot, PCR, and FISH, which are better at finding the stealthy spirochetes (spiral-shaped bacteria that are noto-riously difficult to detect) that cause Lyme disease.

Western blot identifies only one strain of Borrelia burgdorferi, typically found in the Northeast, but there are literally dozens of strains that can cause the disease. His results came back clearly posi-tive. Getting a clear diagnosis started him on a path toward healing. With Alyssa's encouragement and support, we began a course of treat-ment that eventually resulted in dramatic improvement, but I knew there was more he could do to heal.

Unfortunately, due to controversy surrounding chronic Lyme disease in the United States (many doctors insist the condition doesn't even exist), I recommended that they look into an innovative treat-ment facility near the Black Forest in Germany, a hotspot for Lyme infections.

Just before the trip, Burke's health took a turn for the worse. His eyes grew so sensitive to light that he had to wear sunglasses indoors. He collapsed in a coffee shop and, as the pain and weakness became more severe, had to use a cane to get around. Alyssa had to push him through Denver International Airport in a wheelchair to catch their flight to Germany.

The German treatment was safe and beneficial, and Alyssa enrolled in the program right alongside Burke. Three weeks later—after an intensive healing immersion that included many specialized antimi-crobial and nutritional therapies thousands of times stronger than what was available in the United States—Burke walked through the airport on their way home without his sunglasses or cane. I continued to treat him once they returned home.

Burke credits his path to health this way: "Thanks in equal parts to Dr. Jill and Alyssa. They saved my life. Alyssa never gave up, and Dr. Jill melds cutting-edge functional medicine and traditional medicine so well." At the time of this writing, Burke skis every season, says he's ninety-five percent better, and is still working on improvement. But the most precious part to me is receiving their Christmas card photo every year and seeing their smiling faces—alongside their two healthy and vibrant children. Yes, restored fertility was a lovely side effect of Alyssa and Burke's incredible effort to overcome his disease.

Relationship Check-up

We all need routine check-ups, like going to the dentist or eye doctor, and relationships are no different. Here are some questions you can ask your partner to check on the health of your current partnership:

- How healthy do you feel our relationship is?
- Do you feel loved by me?
- Is there anything I no longer do that you miss?
- How connected do you feel in this relationship?
- Do we spend enough quality time together?
- Is there anything I can do that would make your life easier?
- Is there anything I do that has been annoying you lately?
- Is there anything that you feel I have been taking for granted lately?
- How could we have more fun together?
- Do you trust me?
- Is there anything you want us to work on?
- Is there anything you feel uncomfortable talking to me about?
- Do you feel safe with me?
- Do you feel fulfilled in our intimate life? If not, what would make you feel more connected?

NEW WHEELS

While my patient was experiencing the loving support of his partner, my illusion of love disappeared right before my eyes and left me with the equivalent of a cracked handheld mirror, reflecting jagged fragments that I barely recognized. In the aftermath of the separation, we tried one more attempt to heal the broken relationship with professional marital counseling.

After getting to know us over several weeks, one afternoon the therapy took a turn I didn't expect.

"Jill," the therapist said, "Has anyone ever hurt you?" I was confused by the question and remained silent, closing my eyes as I sometimes do to go inside where it felt warm and safe and I could shut out the world. What happened next I now understand, but at the time I had no language or context to make sense of it. My body started trembling and I witnessed myself falling apart, literally beginning to sob and wail like a child. I remember thinking, *How strange! Please pull yourself together, Jill. This is ridiculous.* But at the same time, I also knew there was no way I could have produced this puzzling reaction on a whim. Whatever was happening to my body, the grief was all-consuming, a somatic memory of trauma, one that I had suppressed from conscious memory my entire life.

As I witnessed my own collapse, I could no longer deny the truth. It wasn't just diagnosable diseases that I was tasked with healing from; I also needed to address trauma. From several traumatic childhood experiences to my severe illnesses as an adult, I'd experienced trauma. When I finally understood that I was no longer that helpless little girl but a grown woman with a voice, I decided to file for divorce. Although my husband was not the one who had caused the original trauma, I allowed myself to be further traumatized by believing I had no choice in what was happening. It was empowering to finally understand why many friends and even my own marriage therapist had encouraged me to act instead of waiting for the inevitable. I had been embracing a helpless victim mentality, born of past trauma, a learned "freeze state" that had colored my childhood. This decisive action held healing power for that little girl who at times in the past did not have a choice. It unlocked the freeze response to which I had become accustomed and gave me license to take action this time, challenging the power the past trauma had over me. Supportive relationships and the power to choose differently and mobilize are powerful medicines to begin healing trauma.

The staggering realization that I had a choice opened up something deep inside me that had been there all along. I found myself very desperately wanting to, of all things, buy a motorcycle, the quintessential representation of freedom and bravery. It was certainly a flow-inducer and dopamine producer, and maybe it would help me learn to love again in a healthy way.

I didn't know much about motorcycles, but I knew enough to know I wanted a German-made bike in brilliant red. And so, at forty years old, I drove down to a nearby dealership that sold BMW and Triumph motorcycles. Mind you, I had never ridden a motorcycle in my life. Did that stop me from walking in the door like I owned the place? Not at all! I browsed around the showroom for ten minutes and something caught my eye at the front end of the store. It was a beautiful dual-sport adventure bike, a BMW GS700, looking sporty and hot, with big black tires, a gorgeous red body, sparkling chrome finishing, and a darling purple coil for suspension that made me smile.

The salesperson demonstrated how to throw my right leg over the seat and sit on the bike while it was still propped up on the kickstand. I sat down on the bike and felt an immediate wave of warmth and excitement wash over me. Some might say it was a whim, but I knew better. I was home. I was in love. Not with the bike particularly but with myself being on the bike—just what I needed. Secretly I had always wanted a motorcycle and to learn to ride on the open road, but no one who I knew owned and rode a motorcycle.

I looked over at the salesperson, cocked my head to the side, and said, "I'll take this one. Can you deliver it? I don't know how to ride. Yet." The shocked salesperson looked at me and said, "Will you need a loan? We've got great options for financing."

"No," I said. "I'll write you a check today."

This decision meant there was no turning back. And I realized that even though this was empowering, there was still a tinge of fear because I had no idea what would happen when I actually got on that bike. But I also knew my decision came from a better place of self-compassion and self-trust. Trusting myself and my intuition was the first step that allowed me the freedom to make better decisions instead of just responding unconsciously. About ten days later, the delivery crew pulled into my condo parking lot with a trailer, opened the back end, and wheeled down my brand-new BMW onto the pavement: my own personal love machine.

Over the next several months I was too busy to take lessons, and the bike sat in my garage. Almost every day I would go out and talk

How to Be Kind to Yourself

Based on my *Think Act Be* podcast interview with Seth J. Gillihan and a follow-up article in *Psychology Today*,[52] here are some things you can to do be kinder to yourself:
- Let your experience be what it is.
- Love yourself. You're doing the best you can.
- Know that there will be difficulties.
- Don't judge how you're dealing with it.
- Love others and seek out friends and family who show you unconditional love

to her: "Hey, girl, we are going to take some beautiful adventures on the open road, you just wait!"

Finally, two months later, I took a motorcycle rider class on a small Honda. I had a blast and was easily able to handle the smaller bike. With my training done, it was time to ride my love machine! With my heart racing in the most pleasant way, I carefully put it in neutral and rolled it backward out of the garage into the street. It was going to be a whole lot of love; when I felt the enormous difference between the small Honda and this BMW, nearly three times the size and weight, I wondered aloud, "What did I get myself into?" Had I made a mistake? But I quickly fired up the sweet-sounding engine and proceeded down the road for my first ride—slowly at first, but then . . . wow! What an exhilarating feeling. As I cranked up the accelerator, I felt the incredible rush of euphoria, the feeling of empowerment and speed and complete freedom in the open air. I was in *love* with myself on this bike and the empowerment I felt. I had always dreamed of this day—a dream that I had pushed deep within me, like other unpleasant emotions, because it didn't fit what I saw as "appropriate" based on my past conditioning. My dear friend Dr. Shelese Pratt said it best one day in regard to both my love for risky adventure and my Highly Sensitive Person, "Jill, you can still be a badass and a delicate flower!"

In some ways, buying a motorcycle was the forty-year-old divorcee version of my cottage cheese incident when I was two. I was sitting in my high chair in the kitchen before church, freshly bathed and wearing my Sunday best with a bib to catch the crumbs of food. I was eating a snack of cottage cheese, one of my favorite foods. As was typical in the Hodel household, my older brother was stirring up mischief, while my younger brother was crying to be changed. Meanwhile I was entertaining myself in the high chair. Always the conscientious one, never causing too much trouble, I politely asked, "More cottage cheese, please?" in a singsong two-year-old voice. "More cottage cheese, please!" I said again, this time pleasant but slightly louder. Over and over, I sang my song asking for a second helping. Finally, I realized that no one was listening and so I dumped what was left in the bowl upside down on top of my head and giggled like mad.

> Buying myself a new motorcycle and learning to ride was a way to rediscover my needs and reconnect with something deeper, something I frequently write on a prescription pad for my patients: "Be kind to yourself!"

Maybe the most important thing was to rediscover what I liked and what I needed. After practicing so long suppressing my needs, I hardly knew what they were anymore. The bike became my secret weapon. Anytime I'm feeling uncertain, I just confidently jump on my BMW, knowing she will bring me into a flow state with the resulting feeling of freedom and creativity and, most of all, love: love for myself and love for life, qualities that are every bit as important to healing as any drug or nutrient.

WORK VS. PLAY

Riding a motorcycle, with no goal other than enjoying the ride, made me realize that maybe it's okay to do things without being productive—that simply being is worthy of love. Now I am learning that I don't need the bike to enjoy the ride; I can create the same feeling sitting in my favorite chair in the morning, reading or praying for others, or just having quiet time to process my own thoughts. Before, if I wasn't producing, I felt guilty, small, insignificant, or without value. I could hardly sit still prior to this new understanding that *being* was just as valuable as *doing*!

I used to get up and go running (often clocking five miles by 6 a.m.) or do an intense workout, then shower, rush off to twelve hours of productivity at my clinic until I got home, grab a bite to eat before I began working again, answer emails, and then study until falling into bed exhausted. Sometimes I dreamt of a quiet evening with a delightful book like I used to do years ago before the pressure and deadlines of medical school robbed me of my ability to relax. Other times I wondered if I had ever truly relaxed.

Reading for leisure and daydreaming felt less valuable than accomplishing something concrete, and I didn't see myself as a daydreamer. My perceived value in myself was based on doing—always doing. Who am I if I stop producing, stop running, and stop meeting the demands of everyone around me? What is left? Do I have any value if I'm not meeting people's needs and answering calls and texts?

I began to feel a desperate need to have times in my life where I stopped going at full throttle all the time, but I worried that if I stopped running, stopped producing and answering messages, stopped having meetings, and stopped meeting everyone's demands that my value would be lost. Without constant whirling, producing, and serving others, would I lose myself? Would I still have a purpose? It felt that if I wasn't constantly doing, I lacked essence. I rarely allowed myself to spend time resting, and the guilt I felt when I did was overwhelming.

Although it may have felt good on a superficial level, this hustle was in fact keeping me away from my healing heart space, the quiet and creative space where my soul loves to dwell. In learning to love myself on the back of a motorcycle, I also learned to do the same while simply sitting and meditating in a quiet place.

But my identity was still wrapped up in doing. I had become known as a person who could always be counted on to fulfill a request, no matter what it took. This fed my ego. I had built my life around helping people in need. But it came at a great cost. I have often pushed too far without adequate rest, and the demands would keep coming. Then the overwhelm would hit and would have to shut out the world. I have been terrible at seeing it coming. I keep on the production treadmill, running until the wave of physical exhaustion crashes over me, slamming me to the floor of life. When that happens, the doctor is out, and I close the door and put out the "Do Not Disturb" sign. Only then can I retreat to the quiet place in my heart and soul where ultimate peace resides.

> I can muster the strength to love, encourage, and inspire only when I have first taken time in my inner sanctuary connecting with what I like to call the Divine Creative.

But despite all I've done to heal in my life, this approach of pushing so hard until I can't help but crash is the antithesis of health and healing. I am learning that it's okay to retreat to my inner sanctuary where I can dip my toes in the fresh water and refresh my soul in the quiet of my inner world; in the peaceful, perfect stillness; in the reverie of daydream where my thoughts are my only companions. It is at these times and in the places of quiet solitude where my greatest strength of wisdom and inspiration come. And now I know that I was created for both—the doing and the being.

If I crowd out the place of sacred silence, I lose the essence of what is me, the best parts of me: the joy I bring to the world, the creativity I bring to my work, the peace that others tell me they feel when they're in my presence. Setting healthy boundaries and protecting this precious place of refreshing is another crucial step on the journey to healing.

Dr. Jill's Self-Compassion Practice: SOUL

As you do the work around healing old trauma and unhealthy patterns in your life, sometimes difficult emotions come up. This practice will remind you how to process these emotions with love and compassion:

- **S**it with the feelings that arise.
- **O**bserve and allow them to be present without judgment.
- **U**se understanding to get curious about the feelings. When might you have first felt this same way?
- **L**ove yourself with deep compassion: be kind to yourself!

MINIONS AND MOLD

I had spent my life fighting. I fought the allergens and toxins on the farm as a little girl, I fought cancer and Crohn's disease in my twenties, and now I was fighting mold and relational toxicity. I knew I was strong and able to overcome, and fighting had been my way of doing things. But clearly it wasn't working. I was tired of fighting. I realized what had worked in the past wasn't working anymore. I needed a new strategy. I needed a visualization that would take me from warring against myself to becoming a compassionate peacemaker and collaborator in healing. I suddenly had an idea! Minions, the little yellow creatures with otherworldly engineering and problem-solving skills from *Despicable Me*! I needed minions, not warriors, to help me heal.

It wasn't easy for my alter ego, Sasha the Warrior Princess, to let go of the fight. I was a fighter—a mild-mannered fighter, perhaps, but a fighter nevertheless. And my favorite opponent was myself. When I was seven years old, trying to learn to play piano, I would get so mad at my hands playing the wrong notes that I would sometimes bite my fingers until they bled. After forty years of fighting for my health and for accolades that made me feel deserving of love, I needed a different approach.

It was time to bring Sasha home from the battlefield, take off her sword and shield, and teach her lessons in love and self-compassion. It was time for happy, little, loving, yellow problem-solvers. Every morning on my walk, I started meditating on these minions, imagining them as helpers in my body, walking along whistling. When they'd come across mold (mycotoxins), they would tell the toxin in a friendly voice, "Let's go!" and escort it gently out of my body. Despite all the advanced detox therapies I was doing, I can honestly say that the day I truly began healing was the day I stopped fighting and started meditating on this peaceful multitude of minions cleansing my body of all toxicity.

One of my colleagues in functional medicine, Conan Shaw, explains it best:

> Finding science plus honoring the spirit equals true healing. You can improve, and even be free of disease by definition, but my patients who don't work to heal their spirit slide back towards disease.

Now, looking back at that time across a pandemic caused by a virus that triggers the body's own immune system to fight so the cytokines produced can end up killing the victim, it makes more sense than ever that we need a different paradigm.

}   **It is clear to me that fighting will**   }
}   **never heal; only love heals.**   }

I shared this with a patient suffering from COVID-19, who was coughing so hard he would vomit. He decided to meditate on soothing his immune response with this self-directed loving compassion. He claimed he began recovering the next day, and a month later he was back skiing thirteen-thousand-foot peaks. He focused on the essential goodness of his natural healing system, loving himself in whatever way he could with his thoughts and intention. This is the healing power of unconditional love—loving-kindness to our own body.

As a community, we're caught up in the fight. We gravitate toward conflict that starts with self-criticism, repeating messages from our parents or others, inflaming wounds around self-hatred or self-judgment, and then lashing out at perceived enemies all around us. Imagine if we could model the healing change and present ourselves to the world with love regardless of choices, appearance, belief, or any other quality. What if we responded to the community around us with honor and respect without judgment? The potential to heal on a global scale is real, but it starts with self-compassion. It starts with loving yourself and then extending this love to others.

"You're perfect just as you are!" Many people don't get to hear these words growing up. They instead hear the din of social media manipulating them through false filters and telling them they are not enough: not tall enough, pretty enough, thin enough, smart enough. We need the message more than ever that we are perfect just as we are. Even more important, as I often say, it's our imperfections that make us more lovable. This is where healing begins: loving ourselves as we are without wishing to change and showing ourselves gentle loving kindness and compassion.

In my experience, the Divine Creative is love, and unconditional love for others comes from a greater awareness that we are spiritual beings having a human experience. No matter how well we heal and overcome disease, we have to come to peace with the fact that we are ultimately terminal, but love is eternal.

THE GREATEST OF THESE IS LOVE

Unconditional love is the greatest medicine. I have staked my entire life on this belief. Our mission statement at Flatiron Functional Medicine reads:

> We believe that you can achieve optimal health regardless of the presence or absence of disease. Building on our philosophy of loving people first, we strive to create an environment filled with hope and healing. As we listen carefully to your concerns, we partner with you to create a personalized treatment plan focused on treating the root cause of an illness and empowering your body to begin the innate healing process.

The process of healing starts with loving acceptance of what is. If we are living in defeat or feeling hopeless, it is more difficult to overcome any challenge. Love is the antidote to hopelessness and, as I learned, is far more effective than fighting. But our culture raises us to be fighters: to fight disease, to fight for our rights, to fight for good.

One of my favorite quotes on love comes from Viktor Frankl in his classic book *Man's Search for Meaning*:

> Love is the only way to grasp another human being in the innermost core of his personality. No one can become fully aware of the very essence of another human being unless he loves him. By his love he is enabled to see the essential traits and features in the beloved person; and even more, he sees that which is potential in him, which is not yet actualized but yet ought to be actualized. Furthermore, by his love, the loving person enables the beloved person to actualize these potentialities. By making him aware of what he can be and of what he should become, he makes these potentialities come true.[45]

TAKING OFF THE MASK

I've always felt like I didn't really belong, kind of like an alien. But I know am not alone. I am certain there are others that must feel just like me. Later in life we may identify with the imposter syndrome, which arises when we're in a role or a career, something we've trained to do to the point of being skilled and even respected for it, yet we feel like we don't have it exactly right.

I still have this feeling sometimes, but I've also learned that we're never ready. What sixteen-year-old is *ready* to have a driver's license? What new parent is *ready* to go home from the hospital with a new baby? Who is *ready* to change their diet? Who leaves the doctor's office with a scary diagnosis feeling like they're ready to face the challenge of healing?

> Most of us rarely feel ready for any significant action in life but the point is to take action regardless of our feeling of readiness.

My siblings and parents are rational, stoic, analytical problem-solvers. And then there's me, a sensitive, intuitive, empathetic, bohemian hippy-dancing kind of girl. I am grateful for inheriting some of these analytical problem-solving skills, but I'm sure I was still in diapers when I felt like I didn't fit in. My mom told me I didn't cry much as a baby. It is possible that even as an infant, I sensed that expressing emotion wasn't something we did in my house.

Instead, I conditioned myself to become smaller, trying to blend in. I spent a lot of time feeling as though I managed my life like the volume knob on the radio, keeping it quieter; I felt that I shouldn't be so loud, so creative, so vibrant, so wild, so rebellious—that I should turn down the volume and fit in, not to be noticed. And maybe, just maybe, if I kept my true self small enough, nobody would notice that

I didn't really belong. There was an element of self-preservation in this, but oh my, was it ever costly to my body and soul.

After decades of hiding my inner alien in many interactions with the world, I finally found the remedy was incredibly simple: I learned to show myself love and compassion instead of judgment. Once I was in the world of medicine, it was even more difficult. Medical school in those days was still driven by its patriarchal history, and during my early years as a practicing doctor lecturing, I wore black pant suits. But I hated pants suits! Did my great-grandma hate having to hide her beautiful brunette hair in her hat every day? I suspect she did. But every day she dressed herself up to blend in with the men around her. Just like me.

The black pants suit was another mask I wore to fit into a male-dominated culture. But it is hard to connect with someone in a mask. Eventually I grew tired of pretending to be something that I wasn't, and I began choosing bright, flowing dresses and jewel-tone sheaths with sparkly heels. The more I modeled authenticity, the more it gave others permission to do the same. The audiences in my lectures grew, and I realized I was connecting at a much deeper level.

LETTING OTHERS IN

As I meditated in my favorite chair one morning, I was interrupted by an irresistible thought: *Go into the bedroom and pick up that book.* Although I had picked it up several times, I had yet to read it. I got up slowly, wrapped my cardigan around me, and walked into the bedroom. *Grace and Grit* is a collaborative work written by Ken Wilber and his wife, Treya Killam Wilber, who succumbed to breast cancer but was profoundly changed and spiritually awakened in the process.

I flipped it open to a seemingly random place about halfway through. What my eyes landed on was so profound—and entirely not random—that it took my breath away. It described the works of psychoanalyst Frederick Levinson in *The Causes and Prevention of Cancer*. Ken wrote:

> [Levinson's] theory is that people are more prone to cancer if, as adults, they have a hard time bonding with other people. Rather they tend to be hyper individualistic, overly self-contained, never asking for help, always trying to do it themselves. Because of this, all the stress that they accumulate cannot be discharged easily by bonding with others, or by asking others for help, or by allowing themselves to depend on anyone. This built-up stress thus has nowhere to go, and if they are genetically primed for cancer, the stress can trigger it.[46]

Treya went on to write, "And I know what's beneath it. Fear. Fear of being dependent. Fear of being rebuffed if I were to ask. Fear of being turned down if I showed my need. Fear of being needy."

I remember how quiet I was as a child, how easy, how undemanding, how uncomplaining. I didn't ask for much. I didn't tell anybody about my problems in school or with my friends. I went to my room where I read books alone. Here is Levinson's point: The precancerous individual will most likely be able to experience intimacy only when caring for someone else. This is safe.

My breath caught in my chest with this eerie correlation to my own life and journey with cancer. Here I was, twenty years later, finally understanding how this responsible, capable, and self-sufficient mask had been my prison, keeping me from deep intimacy and letting love in. All I had to do was look back at the types of relationships I had had and the choices I had made, subconsciously choosing men who couldn't truly show up precisely so that I would not have to take off my mask and allow them in.

But I was finally learning to open the doors of my heart. Just a few weeks earlier, I had spent an adrenaline-filled day with a documentary film crew climbing another mountain to capture the experience I'd had on the Third Flatiron. Due to an interview that afternoon, I left slightly earlier than the rest of the crew, so I said my goodbyes, gave everyone hugs, and walked down the mountain alone. Throughout the climb and the experience of that day, I had been completely surrounded by an amazingly supportive and loving team. On the way down the trail, however, I began shaking uncontrollably and felt a bone-chilling coldness. I couldn't get warm. My teeth were chattering, my body trembled uncontrollably, and I knew I was going into a state of shock from hypoglycemia. I continued trembling the entire twenty-minute drive home, and as I walked through the door, I started sobbing uncontrollably. A combination of low blood sugar and the intense experience of rock climbing had hit me hard.

But unlike my younger years, when I would have pretended everything was fine and suppressed the intensity of the day, later that night, when my boyfriend came over, I allowed him to sit me down in my favorite chair, cover me with a warm quilt, and cook dinner for me. I understood that I was still healing my inner little girl, and the best way to do that was by resting and allowing someone to take care of me.

Despite this newfound understanding, the moment I sat down in that chair, I felt an immense ocean of sadness and grief well up inside so strongly that it felt like it was going to drown me. I recognize that this was one of the main reasons I resisted allowing someone to care for me for so many years. The vulnerability that popped up when I allowed myself to rest or be cared for brought with it such an intense wave of grief that I could hardly sit still. It took every ounce of willpower to sit there and not jump up and help my boyfriend make dinner. But I knew that allowing myself to be cared for is where healing resided for those of us used to doing everything for ourselves.

For so long it felt easier to pretend I was strong and capable instead of showing my needs, to be the one others relied on. It was easier than acknowledging the natural vulnerability of being human by letting someone in and running the risk of shattering the carefully crafted image of superwoman.

I realized then that it was no accident I had picked up *Grace and Grit* that morning and opened to the exact page that described parts of my life experience more accurately than I ever could have done. I felt a warm tear slide down my cheek and I whispered softly to myself, "Oh sweetheart, you're so brave and so strong, and it's okay to let others in. This is the path to healing; this is the way to finally allow love in. It's safe now. You can let them love you. You can love you."

Warmth returned. I held both hands over my heart and thanked God for the beautiful living force it possessed, the ability to dance and love, and for all the challenges that set me up so perfectly for whatever tomorrow brings. And with a soft smile, I got up and walked to sit down at the table for one of the most beautiful, unconditionally loving, and healing dinners I'd ever enjoyed.

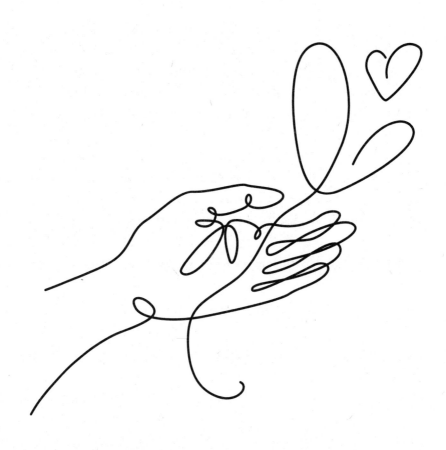

EPILOGUE

Whatever Tomorrow Brings

Our painful experiences aren't a liability—they're a gift.
They give us perspective and meaning, an opportunity
to find our unique purpose and strength.
—Edith Eger, Holocaust survivor
and author of *The Gift.*

WHATEVER TOMORROW BRINGS

As I was finishing this manuscript with deadlines rapidly approaching, I decided to take some time off to write and refresh my weary soul on the beautiful beaches of Hawaii. A few days before I planned to leave for my trip, my sweet puppy, Mario, began to rapidly decline in health, and I could tell he was suffering. The night before I took him into my vet, my intuition knew. He was dying. It broke my heart, but I stayed up all night holding him when he would cry and patiently making him as comfortable as possible. I carried him into the vet the next morning when they opened at 8 a.m. and left him there to work into her packed schedule. I had just walked back into my office and the phone rang, not twenty minutes later. Liv, my vet, was on the line. "Jill," she said, "Mario is in pain and has a severe bladder obstruction. I don't know if we can do surgery. . . ." She paused. I could tell she was holding back from what she really wanted to say, but I already knew. I choked back a sob. "Liv," I said, "it's okay. He's had a long, beautiful life, and I am ready to let him go. I don't want him to suffer any longer." She responded quickly, "Okay. Would you like to come back right now?" I sobbed, "Yes," and hung up the phone, weeping.

My intuition had already told me. I was grateful to have had the previous night holding him, giving him all the love and tenderness I could in his last hours. But I had never done this before. I had never had to say goodbye to a precious companion, almost closer to me and certainly more loyal than any human. As I held him in my arms and watched him take his last breath, I let the emotions flow, both gratitude and sadness mixing with the tears that soaked my face. Life keeps moving on, loved ones come and go, and life will continue bringing us challenges. My old way, the warrior's way, would have been to resist the emotion. Instead, I let myself become soft and vulnerable, allowing it all to flow. Strength is important, yes, but a soft and surrendered strength holds the key to overcoming the obstacles of life and finding meaning and purpose in the process.

I almost didn't go on the trip to Hawaii, but at the last minute I decided I really needed to get away and trust that my other pup, Ravi, would be well taken care of while I was gone. I got on a nonstop flight on Christmas day, and it was only after boarding the plane that my body relaxed and sunk into the seat with anticipation of a vacation. Little did I know that in the last hours of 2021, I would experience another tragedy that would absolutely shock me to the core and change the trajectory of my beloved community forever.

I was able to balance writing with letting go of the workload. I woke up without an alarm, snorkeled in the ocean, climbed volcanoes, and enjoyed the lush tropical shores and black volcanic rock, bamboo forests, tropical birds, and even some of the best coffee Hawaii has to offer. Toward the end of the week, I went hiking at 9,000 feet in a place refreshingly without cell service, when I finally got a frantic message from my office manager stating that deadly wildfires were raging, driven by hurricane-like gusts of wind right near my home and office. She said my neighborhood was evacuating but assured me that Ravi was okay and was being taken to her home just north of the fires. My mind could hardly grasp what was going on. Fires? On December 30, a mile above sea level in Colorado where there would normally be snowdrifts and ice? And my home was being evacuated? And fires burning all around my office building?

I debated whether to immediately get on the next flight home or just wait to see what happened. Once I turned on the news, I saw clips of fires engulfing entire neighborhoods right next to my home and office. I could hardly believe what I was seeing. The Marshall Fire ended up being the worst natural disaster in the history of Colorado, destroying nearly a thousand residential homes and even more businesses in a matter of hours. I watched until I finally went to bed and slept fitfully. I had to surrender, to practice everything I had learned in overcoming obstacles and hardship, to trust that I would be okay no matter the outcome. I went to sleep that night knowing I might wake up without a home or office.

On the flight home, I felt a familiar feeling. Overcoming obstacles breaks us out of our routine, out of our "trance," and forces us to live in the present moment (that is all we really have anyway, and certainly the present is the only place we can do anything about it). Our world is changing, the warming planet and a global economy are spreading environmental illness, and population density allows disasters like fires and illness to impact enormous numbers of people. But within the hardship there will always be opportunities for all of us to become stronger and more resilient. I arrived home on New Year's Day to ash and rubble and the smell of smoke heavy in the air. Fortunately, both my home and office, although smoke damaged, were still standing.

The struggle doesn't end, but our choice to remain soft and open allows us to meet obstacles with grace and to receive their gifts. Vulnerability comes from the Latin root *vulnus* or "wound" and really means "to carry a wound gracefully."

> None of us are without wounds.
> But may we each grow in grace to
> carry them and believe that we can
> overcome whatever comes our way.

Two days after returning home, with the wisps and strong smell of smoke still lingering all around and the blackened ash where there used to stand entire neighborhoods, I gathered my staff together in the office, still without heat or water, to pray for our community and to begin organizing relief efforts. In that moment, as a tear of gratitude rolled down my cheek, I noticed we were all a little closer, a little bit stronger, with more grace and gratitude and looking for ways we could help those who had lost everything. The ash had hardly settled, but it was already happening.

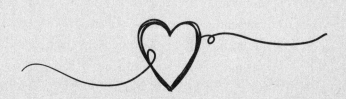

Although you've reached the end of this book, there are more chapters being written for each of us. As you continue your personal journey of transformation and healing, I am here to support you each step of the way.

Please visit my Resources Page for more information and to become part of my vibrant community. Together we will experience unexpected miracles! www.ReadUnexpected.com/Resources.

You are loved ♥
Dr. Jill

Scan here for more resources.

Notes

1 Brené Brown, *Daring Greatly* (New York: Avery, 2015)

2 "What is Functional Medicine?" The Institute for Functional Medicine, https://www.ifm.org/functional-medicine/

3 "Body Burden: The Pollution in Newborns," Environmental Working Group, June 14, 2005, https://www.ewg.org/research/body-burden-pollution-newborns.

4 "Hey Mami!," Dr. Christine Maren, https://www.heymami.com

5 "Highly Sensitive Person," *Psychology Today*, https://www.psychologytoday.com/us/basics/highly-sensitive-person.

6 James G. Wilson, "Environmental Chemicals," in *General Principles and Etiology*, ed. James G. Wilson and F. Clarke Fraser (New York: Springer, 1977), 357–85.

7 R. J. Haworth, E. E. MacFayden, and M. M. Ferguson, "Food Intolerance in Patients with Oro-Facial Granulomatosis," *Human Nutrition*. Applied Nutrition 40, no. 6 (December 1986): 447–56.

8 "Symptoms of Celiac Disease (Celiac Spruce)," Stanford Health Care, https://stanfordhealthcare.org/medical-conditions/digestion-and-metabolic-health/celiac-disease/symptoms.html.

9 Tasha Stoiber, "What Are Parabens, and Why Don't They Belong in Cosmetics?," Environmental Working Group, April 9, 2019, https://www.ewg.org/what-are-parabens.

10 Chuiyan Mo, "Phthalate Regulations in the European Union: An Overview," Compliance Gate, August 14, 2020, https://www.compliancegate.com/phthalate-regulations-european-union/.

11 Seema Patel, "Fragrance Compounds: The Wolves in Sheep's Clothings," *Medical Hypotheses* 102 (May 2017): 106–11.

12 Anne-Laure Demierre, Ronald Peter, Aurelia Oberli, and Martine Bourqui-Pittet, "Dermal Penetration of Bisphenol A in Human Skin Contributes Marginally to Total Exposure," *Toxicology Letters* 213, no. 3 (September 2012): 305–8.

13 O. Al-Dayel, J. Hefne, and T. Al-Ajyan "Human Exposure to Heavy Metals from Cosmetics," *Oriental Journal of Chemistry* 27, no. 1 (2011): 1–11.

14 "34 Great Scientists Who Were Committed Christians," *Famous Scientists*, https://www.famousscientists.org/great-scientists-christians/.

15 Bonnie Azab Powell, "'Explore as Much as We Can': Nobel Prize Winner Charles Townes on Evolution, Intelligent Design, and the Meaning of Life," *UC Berkeley News*, June 17, 2005, https://www.berkeley.edu/news/media/releases/2005/06/17_townes.shtml.

16 "Cleve Tinsley IV: Black Protestant Have a Unique Relationship with Science," *Faith and Leadership*, October 15, 2019, https://faithandleadership.com/cleve-tinsley-iv-black-protestants-have-unique-relationship-science.

17 Benjamin Buemann and Kerstin Uvnäs-Moberg, "Oxytocin May Have a Therapeutical Potential against Cardiovascular Disease. Possible Pharmaceutical and Behavioral Approaches," *Medical Hypotheses* 138 (May 2020): 10597, https://doi.org/10.1016/j.mehy.2020.109597.

18 Yu-Feng Wang, "Center Role of the Oxytocin-Secreting System in Neuroendocrine-Immune Network Revisited," ResearchGate, February 2016, https://www.researchgate.net/publication/311562266_Center_Role_of_the_Oxytocin-Secreting_System_in_Neuroendocrine-Immune_Network_Revisited.

19 A. W. Kneier and L. Temoshok, "Repressive Coping Reactions in Patients with Malignant Melanoma as Compared to Cardiovas-

cular Disease Patients," *Journal of Psychosomatic Research* 28, no. 2 (1984):145–55, DOI: 10.1016/0022-3999(84)90008-4.

20 Gabor Maté, *When the Body Says No* (Hoboken: Wiley, 2011)

21 Jon Tollefson and Erin Hodgson, "Cancellation of Furadan (carbofuran) for Crops Use," *Integrated Crop Management News*, Iowa State University, June 2, 2009, https://crops.extension.iastate.edu/cropnews/2009/06/cancellation-furadan-carbofuran-crops-use.

22 Yuka Yoneda, "Common Herbicide Causes a Sex Change in Frogs," *In Habitat*, March 3, 2010, https://inhabitat.com/common-herbicide-causes-a-sex-change-in-frogs/atrazine-usage-in-the-us/.

23 https://onlinelibrary.wiley.com/doi/abs/10.1002/bdrb.20110

24 S. Greer and Tina Morris, "Psychological Attributes of Women Who Develop Breast Cancer: A Controlled Study," *Journal of Psychosomatic Research* 19, no. 2 (April 1975): 147–53, https://doi.org/10.1016/0022-3999(75)90062-8.

25 Susan Cain, *Bittersweet* (New York: Crown, 2022)

26 Alessio Fasano, "Zonulin, Regulation of Tight Junctions, and Autoimmune Diseases," *Annals of the New York Academy of Sciences* 1258, no. 1 (July 2012): 25–33, https://doi.org/10.1111/j.1749-6632.2012.06538.x.

27 Gilad Halpert and Yehuda Shoenfeld, "SARS-CoV-2, the Autoimmune Virus," *Autoimmunity Reviews* 19, no. 12 (December 2020): 102695, https://doi.org/10.1016/j.autrev.2020.102695.

28 Jin Yang, Kai-xiong Liu, Jie-ming Qu, and Xiao-dan Wang, "The Changes Induced by Cyclophosphamide in Intestinal Barrier and Microflora in Mice," *European Journal of Pharmacology* 714, nos. 1–3 (August 2013): 120–24, https://doi.org/10.1016/j.ejphar.2013.06.006.

29 David L. Suskind et al., "The Specific Carbohydrate Diet and Diet Modification as Induction Therapy for Pediatric Crohn's Disease: A Randomized Diet Controlled Trial," *Nutrients* 12, no. 12 (2020): 3749, https://doi.org/10.3390/nu12123749.

30 Jeffrey Bland, *The Disease Delusion* (New York: Harper Wave, 2014)

31 Steven Kotler, *The Art of Impossible* (New York: Harper Wave, 2021)

32 Alison Gopnik et al., "Changes in Cognitive Flexibility and Hypothesis Search across Human Life History from Childhood to Adolescence to Adulthood," *PNAS* 114, no. 30 (July 25, 2017): 7892–99, https://www.pnas.org/doi/pdf/10.1073/pnas.1700811114.

33 Edith Heard and Robert A. Martienssen, "Transgenerational Epigenetic Inheritance: Mythos and Mechanicsms," *Cell* 157, no. 1 (March 2014): P95–109, https://doi.org/10.1016/j.cell.2014.02.045.

34 R. Ponnusamy, A. M. Poulos, and M. S. Fanselow, "Amygdala-Dependent and Amygdala-Independent Pathways for Contextual Fear Conditioning," *Neuroscience* 147, no. 4 (July 2007): 919–27, https://doi.org/10.1016/j.neuroscience.2007.04.026.

35 "Climate Change Indicators: Lyme Disease," United States Environmental Protection Agency, https://www.epa.gov/climate-indicators/climate-change-indicators-lyme-disease#ref4.

36 https://www.ncbi.nlm.nih.gov/pmc/articles/PMC4740122/

37 David Francis and Henry Hengeveld, "Extreme Weather and Climate Change," Minister of Supply and Services, 1998, https://meteor.geol.iastate.edu/gccourse/history/trends/ExtremeWxClim.pdf.

38 "Mold and Moisture." *Architect*, March 22, 2007. https://www.architectmagazine.com/design/mold-and-moisture_o.

39 Cheryl F. Harding et al., "Mold Inhalation Causes Innate Immune Activation, Neural, Cognitive and Emotional Dysfunction," *Brain, Behavior, and Immunity* 87 (July 2020): 218–28, https://doi.org/10.1016/j.bbi.2019.11.006.

40 Claudia S. Miller and Nicholas A. Ashford, "Possible Mechanisms for Multiple Chemical Sensitivity: The Limbic System and Others," National Library of Medicine, https://www.ncbi.nlm.nih.gov/books/NBK234808/.

41 Janice K. Kiecolt-Glaser et al., "Marital Quality, Marital Disruption, and Immune Function," *Psychosomatic Medicine* 49, no. 1 (January/February 1987): 13–34, http://pni.osumc.edu/stressandhealth/KG%20Publications%20(pdf)/018.pdf.

42 Panksepp, Jaak. *Affective Neuroscience: The Foundations of Human*

and Animal Emotions: Series in Affective Science. (New York: Oxford University Press, 2004).

43 Panksepp, pg. 263

44 C. Rogers, "The Interpersonal Relationship: The Core of Guidance," in *Interpersonal Growth and Self Actualization in Groups,* ed. Raymond M. Maslowski and Lewis B. Morgan, 176–89 (New York: Arno Press, 1973).

45 Viktor Frankl, *Man's Search for Meaning* (New York: Pocket Books, 15th Printing Edition, May 2, 200)

46 Ken Wilber and Treya Killam Wilber, *Grace and Grit* (Boulder, CO: Shambhala , 2000), pg. 236-37.

47 "What is Functional Medicine?" The Institute for Functional Medicine, https://www.ifm.org/functional-medicine/

48 "Debunking the Myth of 'Leaky Gut Syndrome,'" Gastrointestinal Society, https://badgut.org/information-centre/a-z-digestive-topics/leaky-gut-syndrome/.

49 Camilleri, Michael. "Leaky Gut: Mechanisms, Measurement and Clinical Implications in Humans." *Gut* 68, no. 8 (2019): 1516–26.

50 Williams Turpin et al., "Increased Intestinal Permeability Is Associated with Later Development of Crohn's Disease," *Gastroenterology* 159, no. 6 (December 2020): P2092–2100.E5, https://doi.org/10.1053/j.gastro.2020.08.005.

51 Leila B. Giron et al., "Plasma Markers of Disrupted Gut Permeability in Severe COVID-19 Patients," *Frontiers in Immunology* 12 (June 2021): 686240, https://doi.org/10.3389/fimmu.2021.686240.

52 Seth J. Gillihan, "How to Be Kind to Yourself Even with a Chronic Illness," *Psychology Today*, January 10, 2020, https://www.psychologytoday.com/us/blog/think-act-be/202001/how-be-kind-yourself-even-chronic-illness.